The Jingfang Case Studies and
Medical Treatises of Dr. Lou Shao-kun

THE JINGFANG CASE STUDIES AND MEDICAL TREATISES OF DR. LOU SHAO-KUN

婁紹昆經方醫案醫話

LOU SHENSHAN

TRANSLATED BY WILL CEURVELS

purple cloud
press

DISCLAIMER

Library of Congress Control Number: 2024915005

Hardcover ISBN-13: 978–1-991081–08-7
Softcover ISBN-13: 978–1-991081–07-0

FRONT COVER ART
Jennifer King
www.jenniferkingstudio.com

COVER DESIGN
Anne-Maree Taranto

INTERIOR DESIGN
Barbara Tada

Published by Purple Cloud Press
purplecouldinstitute.com
purplecloudpress@gmail.com

Purple Cloud Vision

Purple Cloud Press was founded on the principle that only by merging theoretical knowledge and practical experience is one able to gain true understanding and grasp the nuances of pertinent writings. Therefore, all publications by Purple Cloud Press are underpinned by this principle of scholar-physician and scholar-practitioner into the following threefold mission;

- To publish the works of the founders of the Purple Cloud Institute and other authors' finished works in the field of Eastern medicine, Asian religions and martial arts,
- To translate original ancient Asian texts into the European languages,
- To commission writings about masters' and teachers' lineage traditions.

Purple Cloud Press incentivizes authors and translators by guaranteeing them a large percentage of the royalties in order to encourage continued translation projects as well as by providing a platform to reach the largest possible readership. Purple Cloud Press strongly believes that this will help make accessible the profundity of treasures previously hidden from the non-Chinese speaking world.

purple cloud
press

Contents

TREATISES ON JĪNGFĀNG MEDICINE

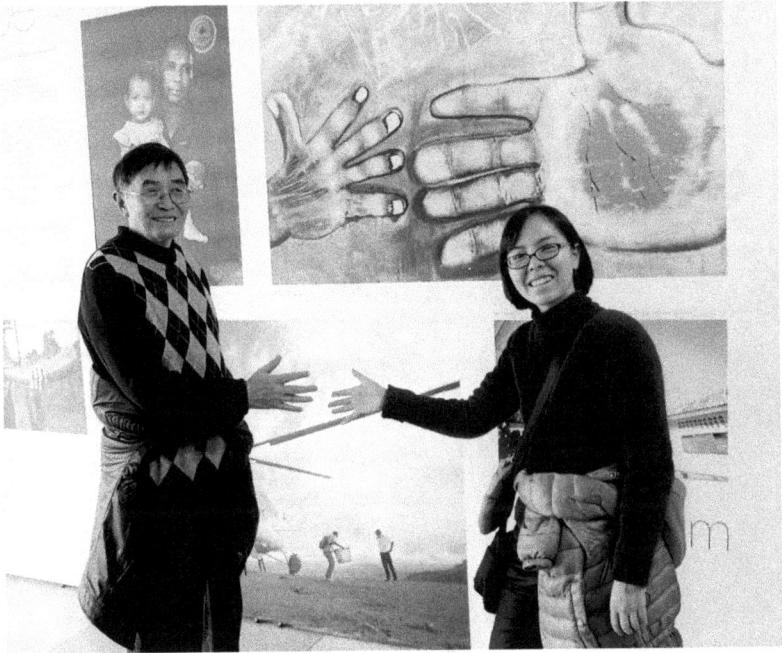
Dr. Lou Shao-kun and his daughter Dr. Lou Shen-shan.

Author's Foreword

DUE TO THE CIRCUMSTANCES of his youth, my father, Lou Shao-kun, had to teach himself Chinese medicine. Despite the difficulties presented by self-study of such a difficult subject, he never tired in his efforts and devoted his entire life to research and study of the *Treatise on Cold Damage* and practice of jīngfāng. His 2012 autobiography *A Life Devoted to Chinese Medicine: One Master Physician's Long Engagement with Jīngfāng* became a bestseller and was widely read not just in Chinese medical circles but in segments of the general public as well. We received many letters from physicians engaging in self-study of Chinese medicine as well as jīngfāng hobbyists requesting that we publish Dr. Lou's case studies and medical treatises.

To this end, I began compiling articles and cases my father had written over the course of his multi-decade career. These writings mostly came from articles he had published online, various lectures he'd given on jīngfāng throughout the country and highlights from *A Life Devoted to Chinese Medicine*. These compiled writings make up the bulk of the "Lou Shao-kun Jīngfāng Series" consisting of *The Jīngfāng Cases and Medical Treatise of Lou Shao-kun* and *Lou Shao-kun: The Jīngfāng Lectures*. *The Jīngfāng Cases and Medical Treatise of Lou Shao-kun* includes my father's personal case studies and details how he combined an internal medicine approach consisting of use of the four examinations, abdominal palpation and jīngfāng formula pattern diagnosis, with an external medicine approach consisting of acupuncture and other modalities to treat various difficult and intractable diseases. The medical treatises included in this book and *The Jīngfāng Lectures* record my father's thoughts and insights from his lifelong research into the *Treatise on Cold Damage* and the *Essential*

Prescriptions of the Golden Cabinet and shed light on his approach to the practice and implementation of jīngfāng medicine. These writings also reflect the clinical experience my father garnered in over forty years of practice, provide insight into the system of clinical practice he developed and detail certain academic investigations of various jīngfāng topics. Importantly, his writings also highlight certain issues and problems currently afflicting the Chinese medical world.

It is my hope that the publication of this book series will serve as a platform through which we can exchange experience in our research and practice of jīngfāng medicine, impart knowledge of jīngfāng to future generations and accelerate the spread of jīngfāng throughout the world.

—Lou Shen-shan
August 15, 2018
Wenzhou, China

Prologue

THE EARLY DECADES OF the twenty-first century were a heady time in China. After two-thousand years of dynastic rule, the great edifice of the Chinese imperial system finally crumbled, and its citizens were faced with an uncertain fate: who would rule their new country and how would it be organized? In the political and ideological vacuum left behind by the dissolution of the Qing Dynasty, ideas became a matter of literal life and death, fortune or famine. In 1912, as the new republic was birthed from the ashes of the imperium, a young Mao Zedong was holed up in a library pouring over the great works of the western liberal tradition—He read Adam Smith's The Wealth of Nations, Darwin's Origin of Species and John Stuart Mill's Utilitarianism. Later, he and his fellow students would found the "New People's Study Society", an organization devoted to the study of new ideas that could guide China on its uncertain path forward. For those of us living at a far remove from revolution and revolt, in a post-modern world suspicious of "absolute truths", it might be difficult to imagine how these revolutionaries invested such a world-historic import in mere ideas, but for these young minds faced with the blank political canvass of a leaderless China, nothing could have been more vital.

Reading through the works of Lou Shao-kun, one is immediately catapulted back into the heady milieu of early twentieth-century China. While a physician by trade, Lou was clearly possessed of a ferocious intellect and his medical treatises are shot through with the fruits of his wide-ranging scholarly exploits. Alongside quotes from the greats of the *kampo* lineage we find references to Marx, Hegel, Lukács, and Lévy-Bruhl. Lou's engagement with ideas was not, however, some frivolous foray, Lou believed like Huang Huang that "conceptual models decide clinical outcomes" and he was of the firm belief that "what the Chinese medicine world needs now is more practitioners...who dare to question, dare to experiment, dare to seek the truth and dare to innovate."

For Lou, Chinese medicine has reached a watershed moment not unlike (nor unrelated to) the upheavals of the Chinese republic in the early twentieth century. In Lou's estimation, the infiltration of a Confucian ethos and praxis into Chinese medicine in the Song dynasty led to an unhealthy preoccupation with abstruse theory and pathomechanism-based diagnosis, at the expense of what Lou saw as the more scientific approach of pre-Song jīngfāng medicine with its emphasis on the clinical reality of symptom and sign presentation. (Lou gives a fascinating account of this process in the essay "Reflections on Abdominal Patterns" included below) In recent years, jīngfāng has seen a resurgence, but according to Lou, "it is still in a formative, inchoate stage — the diagnostic system is not complete and it cannot yet be applied in all situations". Thus, our generation must shoulder the gargantuan, once-in-a-millennium task of revitalizing and perfecting this classical system that by lucky trick of history, snuck out from the behind the slumbering giant of Confucian scholasticism and has come to define new horizons of Chinese medical potential in recent decades.

For his part, Lou believes that one key to the revitalization of jīngfāng medicine is a serious engagement with the clinical experience and medical ideologies of the Japanese kampo lineage. Lou read Japanese fluently, and his works are peppered with references to the works of kampo masters like Yoshimasu, Ōtsuka, Fujihara, Yakazu, Kyūshin and many others. One of the greatest lessons Lou derived from the Japanese was an emphasis on abdominal palpation and diagnosis. Lou often quotes Yumoto Kyūshin, who stated, "The abdomen is the source of life itself and is thus at the root of all disease. As such, abdominal palpation is an indispensable aspect of diagnosis" and Tōdō Yoshimasu, who similarly opined that "one should not prescribe a formula if the abdominal pattern is unclear". For Lou, abdominal palpation is a simpler and more direct form of diagnosis than pulse, which he worries is too mediated by theoretical inference. Abdominal palpation, by contrast, can directly yield "abdominal patterns", which in turn form important constituents of formula patterns, the key to diagnosis in the jīngfāng system. Reading through the case studies in this volume, one gets a clear sense of the deciding role that abdominal palpation plays in Lou's diagnostic process. These studies will be an indispensable learning tool for western students of jīngfāng, teaching us how to integrate abdominal diagnosis or fukushin into our intake and how the results of palpatory findings can inform our diagnosis and treatment approach.

While Lou encouraged Chinese physicians to learn from the Japanese, he still retained a critical stance towards their ideologies. He called Tōdō Yoshimasu's insistence on pure formula pattern diagnosis with no recourse to theory an "over-correction", but admitted that "if not for this over-correction, jīngfāng would never have broken free from the spell of *Inner Canon* mechanism theory and returned to a diagnosis and treatment system truly centered around the *Treatise*". Despite his critical attitude towards Yoshimasu, it is clear that formula pattern correspondence is the keystone element of Lou's clinical approach. As Lou describes, formula pattern diagnosis requires a certain amount of faith and discipline and a kind of "unlearning" of the pre-occupation with mechanisms and etiology of disease we all learn in school. Lou recounts a case in which he is questioned by a patient for palpating his abdomen when he complained of pain in his shoulder—yet, his unrelenting commitment to formula pattern diagnosis and eventual prescription of Tao He Cheng Qi Tang in that case ultimately yields an unexpected and miraculous result.

However, Lou also describes exceptions to the rule, cases in which only mechanism-based diagnosis and treatment resolved a patient's condition. We can trace this dialectical struggle between the theoretical abstraction of mechanism-based *"Inner Canon"* medicine and the practical, empirical rigor of the *Treatise's* formula pattern diagnosis throughout Dr. Lou's work. To Lou, this was an unresolved problem: to what degree should theory intervene in the "primitive mentality" (野性思維, a term borrowed from Lévy-Bruhl) of pattern correspondence? As in any dialectic, out of the synthesis of opposites, the interplay of theory and practice, a new truth will emerge. In Lou's work we see him labor with a rigorous and indomitable intellectual fervor to uncover these ultimate medical truths out of the dialectical struggle of the clinical encounter. His studies and treatises provide inspiration to this new generation to "dare to question, dare to experiment, and dare to innovate" and "while steeped in the classics, seek truth from facts".

—Will Ceurvels
Taiwan 2024

THE JĪNGFĀNG CASE STUDIES

Typhoid Fever Treated with Chai Hu Gui Zhi Tang

ZHOU JUN, 28 YEARS, MALE

FIRST VISIT: October 9th, 1996

A robust, self-possessed young man comes walking into the clinic. His somewhat pallid complexion and apathetic expression seem to indicate slight fatigue.

DOCTOR: What can I help you with?

PATIENT: I've got a persistent fever that still hasn't gone away after fifty days as an inpatient in the local hospital. Last time I checked, my temperature was 38.8°C and while at the hospital I was diagnosed with typhoid fever. (Listening examination: His voice is slightly hoarse.)

THOUGHT PROCESS: In Chinese medicine, there are two forms of heat effusion: a subjective feeling of heat effusion in the patient and independently observed heat effusion. Independent observations of heat effusion include readings on a thermometer or a feeling of heat upon palpation as observed by a doctor. The thermometer reading confirms that this patient indeed is displaying heat effusion.

DOCTOR: Can you tell me how the fever started?

PATIENT: I've been living abroad in Spain for the last seven years and I came back to China for the first time this year to visit family. On my flight back to China on the afternoon of August 16th, I began experiencing some discomfort: I developed a slight headache, felt averse to cold,

11

and lost my appetite. I didn't take my temperature at that time, but later that night, I began to feel very cold. By the time we got to the Shanghai airport, I was in pretty bad shape. On my flight back to Wenzhou from Shanghai, I felt feverish, averse to cold, fatigued and had a headache, pain in my lower back, and had completely lost my appetite. I felt terribly uncomfortable. When I finally got home, my temperature was 38.0°C. It wasn't a high fever, but I felt very uncomfortable, so I went to a local hospital. Blood tests showed that I had a reduced white blood cell count, and after a few more days of examinations and observation, I was diagnosed with typhoid fever and admitted as an inpatient. During my time as an inpatient, my fever went as high as 40°C. This week, my temperature has been steady at around 38.0°C. I still have a lot of full-body discomfort.

DOCTOR: Can I see your hospital record?

PATIENT: Here it is, but this is a copy. (The patient had indeed been diagnosed with typhoid fever and treated according to standard western medical protocol)

THOUGHT PROCESS: Typhoid fever corresponds to what the ancients once called "cold damage" or "warm epidemic". The *Treatise on Cold Damage* (傷寒論) used typhoid fever and other related febrile illnesses as models of disease from which common patterns of pathophysiological responses and generalized approaches to treatment based upon such responses could be deduced.

DOCTOR: What symptoms are you currently experiencing?

PATIENT: I have a headache, I feel hot and agitated, and wind and cold make me feel uncomfortable. Even now, while wearing all these layers, the wind and cold still make me uncomfortable. I feel a lot of discomfort in the area below my ribs and the western doctors believe it's due to an enlarged spleen and liver.

THOUGHT PROCESS: In the Chinese medical intake, the first question is always regarding "aversion to cold or heat". Asking about aversion to cold or heat is important as it can alert the practitioner to the presence of external contraction. Fifty days ago, the patient suddenly developed a fever and, yet, felt averse to cold—a case of concomitant heat effusion and aversion to cold—this is an important indicator of tàiyáng disease. Yet, what makes this case a bit abnormal is that the patient still suffers from headache, heat effusion, aversion to cold, and other tàiyáng disease symptoms after a fifty-day hospital stay during which he ran a continual fever. That being said, the six-conformation pattern identification model used in the *Treatise on Cold Damage* primarily focuses on the pulse and pattern presentation in the current moment of an externally contracted febrile disease progression—it is a study of common, generalizable patterns of pathophysiological responses and, as such, is less concerned with the specific number of days the illness has transpired. The next step in questioning is to ascertain specific information about the nature of the patient's concomitant heat effusion and aversion to cold.

DOCTOR: Do the heat effusion and aversion to cold occur simultaneously?

PATIENT: Sometimes they occur simultaneously and sometimes I'll alternate feeling cold or hot. I can alternate between feeling hot and cold several times throughout the course of a day. That being said, there doesn't seem to be any noticeable change in my body temperature from the morning to the afternoon, or from daytime to nighttime. I seem to hover around 38.5°C.

THOUGHT PROCESS: The patient's simultaneous aversion to cold and heat effusion is equivalent to the "aversion to cold with heat effusion" symptomatology included in the symptom pattern for tàiyáng disease in the *Treatise on Cold Damage*, while the alternating aversion to cold and heat effusion corresponds to "alternating cold and heat", an important diagnostic indicator of shàoyáng disease. Given the patient's simultaneous aversion to cold and heat effusion, alternating aversion to cold and heat effusion, and distention and fullness under the ribs, this is clearly a case of tàiyáng shàoyáng dragover disease[1]. The head is the confluence of the yáng and all yáng conformations can display headache, so the nature and position of the headache must be ascertained.

DOCTOR: Where is the pain in your head? Do you feel any other sensations besides pain? Do you feel any abnormal sensations in the nape of your neck and the back of your head?

PATIENT: The pain is mainly on the sides and back of my head, as well as the nape of my neck. I also feel a bit dizzy. When I first fell ill, my neck and back felt stiff and contracted—I actually thought it might be meningitis. That feeling of stiffness went away later on during my hospital stay.

SUMMARY OF FOUR EXAMINATIONS

The patient's illness stemmed from being infected with pestilence qì. Initially, the patient presented with aversion to cold, heat effusion, and headache and spent fifty days as an inpatient in a western medical hospital. Because his fever failed to abate after western medical treatment, the patient sought Chinese medical treatment.

CURRENT SYMPTOMS: Strong aversion to cold, aversion to wind, heat effusion, alternating aversion to cold and heat effusion, sweating, bitterness in the mouth, throat pain, dizziness, temporoparietal headache, and soreness and pain in the joints.

---

[1] On Cold Damage distinguishes two kinds of multiple-conformation diseases: dragover disease and combination disease. In combination disease, symptoms and signs from both conformations appear at the same time. In dragover disease, the patient first exhibits symptoms and signs of one conformation, then symptoms and signs from another conformation appear before those of the first conformation have resolved. In this case, the patient first exhibited symptoms of tàiyáng disease (simultaneous heat effusion and cold aversion, headache, back pain etc.) and then later also developed symptoms of shàoyáng disease (alternating heat effusion and cold aversion, distention and fullness under the ribs) while still retaining the tàiyáng disease symptoms.

TONGUE: Pale red with a thin, pale yellow coating.

PULSE: Floating, wiry, and slightly rapid. (82bpm, 38.8°C)

ABDOMINAL PALPATION: Rigidity of the rectus abdominis, uncomfortable fullness below the ribs, and substernal tightness.

PATTERN: Tàiyáng shàoyáng dragover disease Chai Hu Gui Zhi Tang pattern

TREATMENT STRATEGY: Harmonize construction and defense, harmonize and resolve the exterior and interior.

ANALYSIS: The patient's illness arose due to being infected with pestilential qì . This pestilential wind-cold toxic evil invaded the fleshly exterior, which led the patient to develop tàiyáng disease. Because the exterior contraction was not resolved in a timely manner, the illness progressed into tàiyáng-shàoyáng dragover disease. The invasion of exterior evil caused defense yáng to become congested, depriving the fleshly exterior of warmth, and leading to aversion to cold. Upright qì rising up to combat the external evil caused heat effusion. In summary, aversion to cold, heat effusion, headache, and sweating are all symptoms associated with the tàiyáng disease Gui Zhi Tang pattern, bitter taste in the mouth, throat pain, and dizziness are the three principal symptoms associated with shàoyáng disease and "alternating cold aversion and heat effusion" and "distention and fullness under the ribs" are classic symptoms of the Xiao Chai Hu Tang pattern. Additionally, substernal tightness is a symptom associated explicitly with the Chai Hu Gui Zhi Tang pattern. The pale tongue with thin, pale yellow coating and the floating, wiry, slightly rapid pulse are all indications of a tàiyáng external contraction pattern with concomitant invasion of evil into the half-exterior half-interior. On the basis of the four examinations, this patient was found to have a presentation consistent with a tàiyáng-shàoyáng dragover disease Chai Hu Gui Zhi Tang pattern.

It should be noted that Chai Hu Gui Zhi Tang can be seen as a tàiyáng-shàoyáng dragover disease OR as an intermediary pattern between Gui Zhi Tang and Xiao Chai Hu Tang. The *Treatise on Cold Damage* considers externally contracted febrile disease in its entire scope and development, analyzing the dynamic process of its progression and dividing that process into six continuous stages (the six conformations). Each conformation disease is then divided into several patterns with both overlapping and distinct features. A formula pattern at once consists of a set of the most common, most archetypal and relatively fixed symptoms, while also representing the dynamic process of disease progression. The essence of "administering treatments according to patterns" is to adjust herbal prescriptions in response to changes in patterns. The fixed nature of patterns is relative, while the dynamic nature of patterns is absolute. There is continuity and overlap between patterns and there are many intermediary stages between patterns. As the formula pattern shifts, so too should the formula prescription.

FORMULA: Chai Hu Gui Zhi Tang: Chaihu 15g, Huangqin 10g, Guizhi 10g, Baishao 12g, Banxia 10g, Dazao 5 pieces, Shengjiang 5 slices, Gancao 10g. (1 packet)

ACUPUNCTURE TREATMENT: Let blood at Taiyang (EX-HN-5) and then cup

RESULT: About a half an hour after bleeding and cupping at Taiyang (EX-HN-5), the patient experienced significant relief from his headache. After one day of herbs, the aversion to cold and heat effusion resolved, the patient's temperature returned to normal, and all other symptoms were significantly improved. The patient requested to be discharged from the hospital and continued taking modified Xiao Chai Hu Tang for another week. After completing that course of herbs, the patient felt better and was able to return to Spain in full health a month later. Five years later, when the patient returned home to visit family, he came back to my clinic to thank me. Looking back on that case, everyone recalled that whole treatment process with wonder.

Chronic Urticaria and Recurrent Colds Treated with Gui Zhi Tang plus Shen Qi Wan

MS. QIAN, 40 YEARS, FEMALE

FIRST VISIT: July 8ᵗʰ, 1995

HISTORY: The patient has suffered from chronic urticaria and recurrent colds for the past five years. She has often sought treatment for these issues, but none of the treatments were effective. Both the urticaria and recurrent colds worsened last winter. Currently, both issues continue to plague her, a fact that has caused her much trouble and concern.

CURRENT: The patient has an emaciated build, a pallid complexion, and complains of aversion to wind, excessive sweating, fatigue, weakness of the limbs, and aversion to air conditioning, electric fans, and cold water. Her mouth feels excessively moist, she produces a lot of saliva, and she complains of cold and pain in her lower back and knees. Her digestion, BMs and sleep are all normal. Her period is often delayed, with scant volume and a purple-black color. The period lasts just one day.

PULSE: Sunken and tight

TONGUE: Engorged, pale red with a thin white coating.

ABDOMINAL PALPATION: Rigidity in the lower abdomen with a pen-width ropy knot present upon palpation.[2]

---

[2] This is a Shen Qi Wan abdominal pattern.

PRESCRIPTION: Gui Zhi Tang + Shen Qi Wan

After taking the formula for two weeks, all symptoms were partially resolved, and the patient was overjoyed. To reinforce the effects of treatment, the patient was advised to take ten grams of Shen Qi Wan pills twice a day. The patient continued to take Shen Qi Wan for three months, after which time she reported that all symptoms had gradually completely resolved. Six years later, the patient reported that the symptoms had never returned.

In Chinese medicine, urticaria is called "wind hives" (風疹) and is believed to be primarily the result of defense yang vacuity and blood vacuity engendering wind. However, in this case, the kidney yang vacuity is quite pronounced. *Spiritual Pivot* (靈樞) Ch.18 states, "construction (qì) emerges from the lower burner", while *Spiritual Pivot* Ch.36 states. "The kidney rules the exterior". Based upon these two statements, I concluded that the urticaria and frequent recurring colds were closely related to the kidney yang vacuity pathology. I prescribed Shen Qi Wan, combined with the defense-construction harmonizing Gui Zhi Tang. This prescription yielded good results and was reinforced using just Shen Qi Wan, after which a complete recovery was achieved.

I have found that for chronic urticaria in children under eight years old, adults over 60, and post-menopausal women, Shen Qi Wan should be the first-choice formula. In children, kidney qì has not fully developed, while in adults over 60 and post-menopausal women, kidney yáng has waned. As such, in both situations the vacuous kidney yáng is unable to engender defense qì. Of course, one should always adhere to pattern identification in clinic and use the formula that matches the pattern, being cognizant of possible deviations in individual cases.

Allergic Rhinitis Treated with
Xiao Qing Long Jia Shi Gao Tang

MR. W, 17 YEARS, MALE (160CM, 40KG)

FIRST VISIT: March 23rd, 2016

CHIEF COMPLAINT: Continuous rhinorrhea subsequent to sneezing for one year.

HISTORY: For the past year, the patient has suffered from nasal congestion, nasal itchiness, paroxysmal sneezing, continuous rhinorrhea subsequent to sneezing, and frequent headache. These symptoms are present year-round, but during the summer they become almost constant when in air-conditioning. The patient was diagnosed with allergic rhinitis by a western medical doctor.

CURRENT: The patient has a gaunt build, and a dark red, oily complexion with acne covering his chin. He sweats easily and his sweat has a strong odor.

PULSE: Thin and tight

TONGUE: Red with a white coating

ABDOMINAL PALPATION: Rectus abdominis rigidity, substernal palpitations, water splash sound upon tapping, and periumbilical palpitations.

PRESCRIPTION: Xiao Qing Long Jia Shi Gao Tang

FORMULA: Sheng Ma Huang 5g, Gui Zhi 10g, Xi Xin 3g, Bai Shao 10g, Ban Xia 10g, Sheng Shi Gao 30g, Gan Jiang 5g, Wu Wei Zi 6g, Gan Cao 5g. (Five packets, one packet per day)

SECOND VISIT: March 29th, 2016

The paroxysmal sneezing and rhinorrhea diminished, excessive sweating, and strong odor resolved, but the patient now complains of vertigo and marked aversion to wind in the legs.

ABDOMINAL PALPATION: Rectus abdominis rigidity, substernal palpitations, water-splash sound upon tapping, and periumbilical palpitations.

FORMULA: Gui Zhi 10g, Fu Ling 20g, Bai Zhu 10g, Wu Wei Zi 6g, Gan Cao 5g. (Six packets, one per day)

Five months later (September 7th, 2016), the patient visited the clinic again and reported that after finishing the herbs, his condition completely resolved, and there had been no recurrence of symptoms. Recently, however, the patient had caught a cold and complained of cough, paroxysmal sneezing, rhinorrhea, headache, sweating, aversion to wind, and heat effusion.

PULSE: Floating and rapid

TONGUE: Red with a white coating

ABDOMINAL PALPATION: Rectus abdominis rigidity.

FORMULA: Gui Zhi 10g, Bai Shao 10g, Sheng Jiang 5 slices, Da Zao 3 pieces, Gan Cao 5g, Hou Pu 10g, Xing Ren 10g. (Three packets, one per day)

CLINICAL INSIGHT

Upon noting the patient complained of long-standing aversion to wind, rhinorrhea subsequent to sneezing, and substernal palpitations accompanied with a splashing water sound upon tapping, my first impression was that the symptomatology resembled a Xiao Qing Long Tang pattern. Yet, there were certain symptoms that didn't exactly fit the pattern, such as the dark red, oily complexion, sweating easily, and the strong odor of the patient's sweat and sebum. After further consideration, I concluded these symptoms were representative of a Ma Huang-Shi Gao-Gan Cao pattern sub-group[3], so, I prescribed Xiao Qing Long Jia Shi Gao Tang and achieved a good result. The indications described in lines associated with Ma Huang formulas tend to note a lack of sweating, however, the Ma Huang-Shi Gao-Gan Cao pattern sub-group can treat heat effusion with sweating. For instance, Ma Huang Gan Cao Xing Ren Shi Gao Tang, which is just the Ma Huang-Shi Gao-Gan Cao sub-group plus Xing Ren is used to treat "panting with sweating" in the *Treatise on Cold Damage*. This kind of sweating differs from the sweating presentation in Gui Zhi Tang insofar as it has a stronger, more malodorous smell.

Some patients will experience dizziness, palpitations, and insomnia after taking formulas that include Ma Huang. These symptoms typically resolve after treatment concludes. In this case, for instance, the Ma Huang formula disrupted the "stable pathological state" of the disease, attacked the interior rheum and led to vertigo. This can be seen as a mìnxuàn[4] reaction that paves the way for the next stage of treatment.

The combination of Ling Gui Wu Wei Gan Cao Tang and Ling Gui Zhu Gan Tang prescribed on the second visit was based on the patient's symptoms. The dark red complexion, aversion to cold in the legs, and periumbilical palpitations correspond to the Ling Gui Wu Wei Gan Cao Tang pattern, and the substernal palpitations and water splash sound on tapping align with the Ling Gui Zhu Gan Tang pattern.

---

[3] The pattern sub-group or 基证 is a concept Dr. Lou borrows from *kampo* theory regarding the *Treatise on Cold Damage* and refers to small pairings of herbs that work in concert to achieve a certain action.

[4] Referring to an exacerbation of symptoms prior to recovery, sometimes translated as "healing crisis".

Chest Oppression Treated with
Ma Huang Tang plus Fu Ling

MR. L, 51 YEARS, MALE (155CM, 75KG)

FIRST VISIT: November 5th, 2000

CHIEF COMPLAINT: Chest oppression for 3 years.

HISTORY: Three years ago, after recovering from cough, fever, and other symptoms of a cold, the patient began experiencing chest oppression, which has never since abated. The patient has traveled far and wide in pursuit of effective treatments but has yet to find a cure. Western medical doctors diagnosed the patient with chronic bronchitis and cardiac dysautonomia.

CURRENT: The patient has a robust, short and overweight build, a dark complexion, and dry skin. He reports infrequent sweating, a feeling of moistness in the mouth, and copious saliva. Additionally, he complains of having to expectorate a large amount of watery phlegm every morning and heavy snoring during sleep. He is a smoker.

PULSE: Full, replete

TONGUE: Pale red with a thick white coating.

ABDOMINAL PALPATION: Palpitations present from below the sternum to the navel; abdominal muscles are tight and not vacuous.

DIAGNOSIS: Ma Huang Tang Jia Fu Ling pattern

FORMULA: Ma Huang 10g (decoct first before adding other herbs), Gui Zhi 10g, Xing Ren 10g, Gan Cao 6g, Fu Ling 15g. (Five packets, one per day)

SECOND VISIT: March 19th

The patient seems noticeably happier. He reports that one hour after his first time taking the herbs, he experienced some agitation and thought he would sweat, but the sweat never materialized. Soon after that, his urinary output increased, with increased volume at each subsequent bathroom trip. He also reported reduced chest oppression during the night and while asleep. He did not experience the same urinary frequency with the second and third packets. After the third packet, his chest oppression reduced further, and he noticed a significant reduction in saliva and watery phlegm. The same formula was prescribed again, but with a lowered dose of Ma Huang.

FORMULA: Ma Huang 6g, Gui Zhi 10g, Xing Ren 10g, Gan Cao 6g, Fu Ling 15g. (Five packets, one packet per day)

On December 5th, 2015, a fellow villager from Yong Qiang brought his grandson into the clinic for treatment. As soon as he arrived, he excitedly greeted me, but I was a bit confused by his warm enthusiasm because I didn't remember who he was. He explained that fifteen years ago, I had cured him of his chest oppression. As he spoke, he produced a prescription from his pocket with scratchy, indistinct characters and handed it to me. The prescription contained five herbs — it was Ma Huang Tang plus Fu Ling. The patient remembered the whole treatment process as if it were yesterday. He said that after taking the second course of herbs, his chest oppression basically disappeared and the morning phlegm was significantly reduced, so he suspended treatment. For those past fifteen years, he had quit smoking and limited how much alcohol he drank, and the chest oppression never recurred. However, he did still cough up some watery phlegm from time to time and he still snored heavily. Upon abdominal palpation, I found that he no longer had palpitations from below the sternum to the umbilicus and the tension in his abdominal muscles was moderate.

CLINICAL INSIGHT

The patient's robust, short and overweight build, dark complexion, tendency to snore, distended, large abdomen and tight, sturdy musculature are all classic indications of a stagnant cold constitution. This constitution responds well to Ma Huang family formulas and Wu Ji San, among other formulas. The patient's dry skin, infrequent sweating, moist mouth, copious saliva, and replete, full pulse were all symptoms of the Ma Huang Tang pattern, while his tendency to expectorate large amounts of watery phlegm in the morning and palpitations below the sternum and navel were symptoms of Ling Gui Zhu Gan Tang and Fu Ling Xing Ren Gan Cao Tang patterns. Additionally, the target of treatment for Gan Cao Ma Huang Tang is "urgent panting and distressed breathing". As such, I opted to prescribe a combination of Ma Huang Tang and Fu Ling Xing Ren Gan Cao Tang. As the above makes evident, a synergistic thought process that takes into account the focus of treatment, constitution, herbal pattern, and formula pattern provides a systematic and reliable approach to treatment.

One hour after his first time taking the herbs, the patient experienced some agitation and thought he would sweat, but the sweat never materialized. Soon after that, his urinary output increased, with increased volume at each subsequent bathroom trip. That same night, the patient's chest oppression was noticeably reduced. This suggests that after taking Ma Huang Tang or some modification of Ma Huang Tang, one of two mechanisms of action may occur in patients: 1.) The evil is dispersed via sweating, 2.) The evil is drained via diuresis. This is consistent with Yusei Enda's (遠田裕正) understanding of the basic mechanism of Ma Huang

Tang. Regarding the mechanism of Ma Huang Tang, Enda said, "(Ma Huang Tang) strengthens the heart's pulsation, increasing the supply of blood to the whole body from the heart. The increased blood flow to the skin and kidneys encourages the elimination of water via these two structures. As for whether the elimination occurs via sweating or urination, this depends on the patient's specific pathophysiological dynamics at the time of ingestion as well as which herbs are paired with Ma Huang.

Cough, Panting and Chest Oppression Treated with Mu Fang Ji Tang Combined with Ting Li Da Zao Xie Fei Tang

---

MS. L, 80 YEARS (152CM, 65KG)

FIRST VISIT: September 9th, 2005

CHIEF COMPLAINT: Cough, asthma, and expectoration of phlegm for 2 years.

HISTORY: Two years ago, the patient was found to have hypertension, heart failure, and Parkinson's disease and was hospitalized several times. Her symptoms were primarily chest oppression, panting, cough with copious phlegm, and severe constipation. Her condition was severe enough that she was unable to live on her own. One year ago, after undergoing surgery at a large hospital for gallstones, she developed pneumonia, which exacerbated her coughing and asthma, and caused the production of copious phlegm that was difficult to expectorate. At times, her condition was so severe that she would have to sit up all night coughing up phlegm, unable to lie flat on her back, which significantly impaired her sleep quality. In the course of a single year, she was hospitalized four times and was listed as in critical condition several times. She didn't want to pass away in the hospital, so she decided to return home and seek Chinese medical treatment.

CURRENT: The patient has a robust build with a short, overweight stature, and a dark red complexion. She appears anxious and fearful and complains of chest oppression, chest fullness, agitation, and dry mouth with desire to drink water. She coughs and pants constantly all day and night and her copious phlegm is yellow, sticky, malodorous, and difficult to expectorate. Additionally, she complains of constipation with bowel movements occurring only once every few days, incontinence, and frequent urination with yellow malodorous urine. Her legs display pitting edema.

PULSE: Tight and replete

TONGUE: Dark red with a thick white coating

ABDOMINAL PALPATION: Substernal hard glomus and tightness, abdominal muscles are tight and not vacuous.

DIAGNOSIS: Mu Fang Ji Tang Pattern and Ting Li Da Zao Xie Fei Tang Pattern

FORMULA: Han Fang Ji 10g, Sheng Shi Gao 100g, Gui Zhi 15g, Dang Shen 10g, Ting Li Zi 15g, Da Zao 10 pieces, Mang Xiao 10g (dissolve in prepared decoction), Fu Ling 30g. (Five packets, one packet per day)

SECOND VISIT: September 21st, 2005

After taking the herbs, the patient passed a large amount of malodorous, sticky, black stools. The frequency of her coughing and panting was noticeably reduced and she was able to expectorate phlegm more smoothly. Additionally, the pitting edema in her legs was reduced and she reported feeling less agitated and hot. There was no change in any of the other symptoms.

PULSE: Tight, replete

TONGUE: Dark red with a thick white coating

ABDOMINAL PALPATION: Substernal hard glomus, abdominal muscles are tight and not vacuous.

Han Fang Ji 10g, Sheng Shi Gao 100g, Gui Zhi 15g, Dang Shen 10g, Ting Li Zi 15g, Da Zao 10 pieces, Mang Xiao 5g (dissolve in prepared decoction), Fu Ling 30g. (Five packets, one per day)

THIRD VISIT: September 27th, 2005

After taking the herbs, the patient continued to pass malodorous, impacted stools two to three times per day. The frequency of coughing and panting was significantly reduced, expectoration of phlegm was smooth, and the phlegm was yellow-white and sticky. Her urine was yellow, and she reported a slight reduction in incontinence. The pitting edema in her legs was also reduced.

PULSE: Sunken and tight

TONGUE: Dark red with a slimy, white coating

ABDOMINAL PALPATION: Substernal hard glomus

FORMULA: Same as the second visit, but the dosage was gradually reduced with the patient taking herbs for two days and then resting for one day. The patient continued taking the medicine until October 30th, at which point the panting, cough, phlegm, and pitting edema all completely resolved, and bowel movements became regular (once every one to two days).

Eight years later, (August 18th, 2013) the patient's daughter brought her to my clinic again for treatment. After suspending treatment in 2005, the patient had remained in good health for five years and didn't take any medicine during that time. In 2010, she had a relapse of symptoms, but because we were out of town and our clinic's address had changed, they were unable to find us and had to seek treatment from another Chinese medical doctor. Unfortunately, that doctor's treatment was ineffective, so, left with no other options, they used the formula that I had previously given the patient. The formula stabilized symptoms to a degree, but then in 2013, her symptoms worsened. After searching around, they were finally able to locate our new address and happily arrived at our clinic.

CURRENT: The patient appears alert but seems fatigued and her complexion is dark and oily. She complains of continuous coughing and panting day and night and copious, sticky, malodorous, yellow phlegm that is difficult to expectorate. She reports having to sit up all night coughing up phlegm and is unable to lie flat on her back, which has had an adverse effect on her sleep quality. She is constipated, with bowel movements occurring once every several days, and she complains of frequent incontinence with yellow, malodorous urine. She has pitting edema in her legs and complains of chest oppression and fullness, abdominal distention and fullness, agitation, dry mouth, and desire to drink water.

PULSE: Tight and replete

TONGUE: Dark red with a thick white coating

ABDOMINAL PALPATION: Substernal hard glomus, abdominal muscles are tight and not vacuous.

Despite the patient's advanced age and the chronic nature of her illness, the symptoms still clearly pointed to a Mu Fang Ji Tang combined with Ting Li Da Zao Xie Fei Tang pattern. I used the same formula as before with some slight modifications. After taking the herbs, her symptoms once again gradually resolved—her coughing, expectoration of phlegm, and pitting edema were reduced, and her bowel movements slowly normalized. After this change in symptoms, I switched her dosage to once every two days. For about 6 months after that, her condition was stable, but then an unfortunate accident occurred: on February 5th of 2014, her caretaker fed her a large amount of milk too quickly, causing her to die of asphyxiation. She enjoyed a long life of 89 years. On March 22nd, 2015, her daughter came to my clinic with insomnia. Reflecting on her mother's treatment, she said, "Ten years ago, my mother was listed in critical condition by a large hospital on multiple occasions, but after receiving treatment from Dr. Lou, she was able to live another 10 years, enjoying a long life of 89 years. All our family, friends and neighbors were absolutely amazed by Dr. Lou's results!"

CLINICAL INSIGHT

Dr. Yue Mei-zhong (岳美中) stated: "In chronic diseases, one should not be too quick to change formulas." While keeping in mind the need to treat to the pattern, it is very important in chronic diseases to keep with a formula and not change it too cavalierly. The treatment process in this case is a prime example of the importance of this treatment principle.

"The "Lung Wilting, Pulmonary Welling-Abscess and Cough with Qi Ascent Disease, Pulse, Pattern and Treatment" chapter in the *Essential Prescriptions of the Golden Cabinet* (金匱要略) states: "When there is pulmonary welling-abscess and an inability to lie flat with panting, Ting Li Da Zao Xie Fei Tang is indicated." Also, "When there is pulmonary welling abscess, fullness and distention in the chest, full-body edema, nasal congestion, rhinorrhea, loss of sense of smell, counterflow cough, qi ascent, wheezing, and congestion, Ting Li Da Zao Xie Fei Tang is indicated." The majority of commentaries interpret "pulmonary welling-abscess" (肺癰, fèi yōng) as referring to a pulmonary abscess, while only a few interpret it as meaning "lung congestion". Recently, Professor Li Jin-yong (李今庸) has also expressed support for its interpretation as "congestion." That being said, the majority of modern textbooks still interpret it as "pulmonary abscess". Clearly, there is a need to reevaluate this interpretation. "

The quote above comes from an essay by Dr. Xu Bing-lang (徐炳琅) called "Analysis and Identification of the term "Lung Welling-Abscess" in the *Essential Prescriptions of the Golden Cabinet*". Putting aside the debate over the correct interpretation of the term, Ting Li Da Zao Xie Fei Tang and its treatment targets, namely, "Panting with inability to lie flat" and "Fullness and distention in the chest, full-body edema...counterflow cough, qi ascent and wheezing with congestion" are all in keeping with the presentation in the case above. This is why Ting Li Da Zao Xie Fei Tang was prescribed. This clearly illustrates how as long as the formula prescribed matches the patient's pattern, the treatment will be efficacious. As for the argument over the true meaning of "Lung Welling-Abscess", it is not really that important from a clinical standpoint.

Throughout the course of my treatment of this patient, I mostly only used Mu Fang Ji Tang combined with Ting Li Da Zao Xie Fei Tang. Why was it that when I prescribed the formula for her, it was effective, but when she took the prescription filled at a different pharmacy the results were just average? I was quite confused by this disparity in efficacy, so I inquired further with the patient's daughter. The daughter said that in those years that they couldn't find my clinic, they had always gotten the prescription filled at the same pharmacy nearby their house. Apparently, the pharmacist said that the dosage of raw Shi Gao in my prescription was too high. He said that in the absence of fever, that high dosage of Shi Gao would be damaging to the patient's stomach qì, not to mention that the patient was over 80-year-old and would be unlikely to withstand such a large dosage for an extended period of time! As a result, during those years, the pharmacist rarely included raw Shi Gao when filling the prescription, and if he did, he would never add more than 30g. This was probably the main reason why the prescription yielded such middling results. Here, we must consider a relevant issue: The Classical formula tradition (經方, jīngfāng) conceptualizes herbs in a way that is quite different from the mainstream approaches seen in modern herbal and formulary textbooks. In the *Treatise on Cold Damage*, when Shi Gao is combined with Ma Huang or Gui Zhi, as in Da Qing Long Tang, Xiao Qing Long Jjia Shi Gao Tang, Yue Bi Tang, Mu Fang Ji Tang, and even Ma

Xing Gan Shi Tang, the primary synergistic action of this combination is diuresis. What's more, it is absolutely essential that the dose of Shi Gao in Mu Fang Ji Tang must be very large. For reference, the dose of Shi Gao in Da Qing Long Tang is "the size of a chicken egg", whereas the dose in Mu Fang Ji Tang is "the size of twelve chicken eggs". This stark comparison makes the massive dose of Shi Gao in Mu Fang Ji Tang abundantly clear. Perhaps, some might ask: Why are you claiming that Ma Xing Gan Shi Tang has a diuretic action? The line describing the symptomatology for Ma Xing Gan Shi Tang in the *Treatise on Cold Damage* (After inducing sweating and the patient presents with sweating and panting, and does not exhibit severe heat effusion, Ma Xing Gan Shi Tang is indicated.) notes that the formula can be used to treat "sweating with panting". In my actual clinical experience, I have found that this formula does not work by inducing sweating or purging to resolve the pathogenic state of sweating and panting. So, what is this formula's actual mechanism of action? Based upon Yusei Enda's (遠田裕正) theory of pathology, "Sweating, purging, and diuresis: Three basic physiological reactions and their synergistic and antagonistic relationships", it is a simple process of elimination to deduce that Ma Xing Gan Shi Tang must resolve "sweating and panting" via diuresis.

Any doctor or patient that personally witnessed this case firsthand would invariably praise the efficaciousness of the jīngfāng pattern identification model. If we could all achieve results like this in clinic, would there really be any reason to worry about people suspecting Chinese medicine of being unscientific?

Tuberculosis Treated with Chai Hu Gui Zhi Tang plus Xiao Xian Xiong Tang

FEMALE, 25 YEARS

The patient had always been in good health, but in the fourth month of her pregnancy, she developed a low fever, paroxysmal cough with blood-tinged phlegm, and excessive fatigue. Of particular note was the fact that the low fever usually came on at dusk. She was found to be acid-fast positive by a local hospital and was diagnosed with Tuberculosis. Because the patient was already five months pregnant and had a history of two previous miscarriages, the family was desperate to ensure the baby was successfully delivered, so the decision was made to assume the risks and take antitubercular medication. However, the low fever and cough with blood-tinged sputum still hadn't resolved after one month of treatment. Sensing the urgency of the situation, the family decided to try Chinese medicine.

FIRST VISIT: March 12^{th,} 2003

The patient is now six months pregnant. She appears gaunt with rosy cheeks and an overall pallid complexion. She reports that even during the hottest days of summer she feels aversion to wind and her arms and legs are cool. Additionally, she complains of agitation, feeling hot, night sweats, and a dry cough with minimal phlegm. Her phlegm is sticky, occasionally blood-tinged, and difficult to expectorate, and she feels a general sense of discomfort in her chest. The patient also reports that she seems to catch colds easily, has a poor appetite, and complains of bitterness in the mouth, dry heaving, and incomplete bowel movements passed once daily. Urine is pale yellow.

TEMPERATURE: 37.6°C

PULSE: Floating, rapid

TONGUE: Thin white coating

ABDOMINAL PALPATION: Fullness and discomfort in right rib-side and chest, substernal pain upon pressing.

Based upon these symptoms, the patient displays both Chai Hu Gui Zhi Tang and Xiao Xian Xiong Tang patterns. I decided to first prescribe Chai Hu Gui Zhi Tang.

FORMULA: Chai Hu 15g, Huang Qin 10g, Dang Shen 15g, Ban Xia 10g, Da Zao 5 pieces, Gan Jiang 5g, Gui Zhi 10g, Bai Shao 10g, Gan Cao 5g. (5 packets)

Additionally, I advised her to continue taking her antitubercular Western medicine, get good rest, eat a balanced diet, and try to engage in activities that promoted relaxation.

After one week of herbs, all symptoms improved, aversion to wind and subjective feeling of heat were noticeably reduced, and appetite improved. However, the patient's temperature remained at 37.5°C and there was no change in her abdominal palpation presentation.

Based upon these symptoms, it was clear that she should be treated with a combination of Xiao Chai Hu Tang and Xiao Xian Xiong Tang.

FORMULA: Chai Hu 10g, Huang Qin 10g, Dang Shen 15g, Ban Xia 10g, Da Zao 5 pieces, Gan Jiang 5g, Gua Lou Pi 10g, Huang Lian 3g, Gan Cao 5g. (Seven packets)

After taking herbs for another week, the patient coughed up a copious amount of yellow, sticky phlegm, after which the feeling of congestion in her chest improved. After continuing to take the herbs for another month or so, the patient's temperature returned to normal, her cough with blood-tinged phlegm disappeared, her abdominal presentation normalized, and the results of her pre-natal tests came back normal.

Subsequently, the patient had a smooth delivery, and the newborn was found to be in good health. An x-ray taken after her delivery indicated that the tubercular lesions had calcified. An x-ray of the newborn's chest taken two months after delivery showed no signs of tuberculosis.

CLINICAL INSIGHT

Four months into the patient's pregnancy, she began experiencing mild heat effusion and suffered from paroxysmal cough with blood-tinged phlegm. Later on, she was found to be acid-test positive and was diagnosed with tuberculosis. Because the patient displayed symptoms consistent with Chai Hu Gui Zhi Tang and Chai Xian Tang, I first prescribed Chai Hu Gui Zhi Tang and then later shifted to Xiao Chai Hu Tang combined with Xiao Xian Xiong Tang. After taking the herbs, she coughed up a copious amount of yellow, sticky phlegm, after which the feeling of congestion in her chest improved. After a month of taking this formula, the patient's temperature returned to normal, her cough with blood disappeared, and her overall health recovered.

Dr. Tan Ci-zhong's (譚次仲) *Methods of Self-Care in Lung Illness* recommends Xiao Jian Zhong Tang as the most important formula for treating tuberculosis and Xiao Ping's (蕭屏) *Self-Healing from Lung Illnesses* also regards Xiao Jian Zhong Tang as a fantastic formula for treating the disease. In stark contrast to Tan and Xiao's approach, Shen Zhong-gui's

(沈仲圭) *Chinese Medical Experience Formula Compendium* argues that the primary treatment strategy for Tuberculosis should be "supplementing yīn with sweet cold". The abandonment of a sweet, cold approach for acrid, warm herbs should be regarded as an exception to the rule, only to be used when there is a deviation in the common presentation in tuberculosis. Unfortunately, Dr. Shen did not offer specifics on the kind of presentation that would merit the use of Xiao Jian Zhong Tang, only saying that it would be a yáng vacuity presentation that occurs extremely infrequently in taxation diseases and that if it did present, then the use of Xiao Jian Zhong Tang would be merited.

Wu Jian-hou (武簡侯), a famed 20th century Chinese doctor from Jiangsu had this to say on the debate: "A neighbor of mine named Xu Ke-ming once recalled to me that as a child he had suffered from "taxation" with cough, lower back pain, and night sweats, which hadn't responded to treatments. He later was prescribed Xiao Jian Zhong Tang by one Liu Xing-bo and made a complete recovery after just a few doses." This indicates that Xiao Jian Zhong Tang is indeed a marvelous formula for the treatment of taxation with yīn vacuity. This case seems to provide further credence to Tan and Xiao's claims, but it is worth noting that it would be quite dangerous to neglect performing differential diagnosis and use Xiao Jian Zhong Tang in all cases of taxation with yīn vacuity. The famed Qing dynasty physician and writer Xu Ling-tai (徐靈胎) cautioned: "Xiao Jian Zhong Tang treats taxation with yīn cold and yáng collapse, which is precisely the opposite of yīn vacuity and effulgent fire. Incompetent doctors that use this formula incorrectly have harmed innumerable patients. Japanese *kampo* practitioner Yumoto Kyūshin (湯本求真) noted: "In years past, I tried using Huang Qi Jian Zhong Tang to treat tuberculosis but met with failure. As such, I thought that even in cases of tuberculosis with yáng vacuity, I could use sweet, cold, yīn supplementing medicinals, but in such cases I once again met with failure. Indeed, I had made the same mistake (of just blindly using one method in all cases) in both instances. As physicians, we must endeavor to rout out all subjective tendencies in our clinical thinking process."

All of the arguments represented above conflate treatment based on disease identification with treatment based on pattern identification. They first make the supposition that the common mechanism in tuberculosis is yīn vacuity, and then go on to argue that cases of taxation with yīn cold and yáng collapse represent an exception to the rule. In the context of Chinese medicine, it is truly laughable to talk about disease diagnosis and treatment in a way that is not centered on the actual presentation of an individual patient. Chinese medicine is individualized medicine and one disease can manifest in a thousand ways in a thousand different individuals. How can these physicians speak of yīn and yáng vacuity before they've even seen the patient? If a doctor harbors presuppositions, they will be liable to prioritize a general conceptual understanding over the actual clinical reality of their patient, which will lead their treatment astray.

Takeaways from this Case

Tuberculosis, or "lung taxation" (肺癆, fèiláo) in ancient Chinese medical parlance, is often thought to be the result of either lung and kidney yīn vacuity, yīn vacuity with effulgent fire, consumption of qì and yīn or simultaneous yīn and yáng vacuity. However, none of these patterns even remotely resembles the pattern that presented in this case. This demonstrates that diagnosis and treatment that targets a disease (as opposed to a formula pattern) is still quite lacking as a viable approach. By contrast, the formula pattern correspondence method employed in jīngfāng medicine provides a clear target of treatment, produces reliable results, and is reproducible.

Patients that have already started a regimen of antitubercular medicine should not suspend treatment without proper consideration. It is safer and more effective to treat tuberculosis with Chinese medicine in combination with Western medicine.

Cerebral Stroke Treated with
Da Chai Hu Tang plus Mu Fang Ji Tang

MR. C, 72 YEARS (175CM, 65KG)

FIRST VISIT: October 23rd, 2015

CHIEF COMPLAINT: Full-body tremors and weakness of the limbs for two months

HISTORY: The patient has had a long-standing fondness for alcohol and has a high tolerance—he could drink ~20oz (13 shots) of báijiǔ (or ~100oz (65 shots) of yellow wine (黃酒) at a time. After falling ill two months ago, he quit drinking. He was diagnosed with "cerebral stroke", "atrial fibrillation" and, "pulmonary edema" among other illnesses by a western medical hospital.

CURRENT: The patient has a dark, sallow complexion and reports having experienced chest oppression and occipital head pain for many years. He has infraorbital edema, lower leg edema, and occasionally drools. He complains of poor sleep quality, daytime drowsiness, leg weakness, and inability to stand on his own. He also reports having well-formed stools that are difficult to pass, 5–6 bowel movements per day, scant, frequent urination with yellow, malodorous urine, and nocturnal urination with up to five bathrooms visits per night.

PULSE: Slippery

TONGUE: Dark red with a moist, glossy coating

ABDOMINAL PALPATION: Tight, replete abdominal muscles, fullness and discomfort in the chest and rib-side, pain upon knocking at the gallbladder, and substernal hard glomus[5].

DIAGNOSIS: Combined Da Chai Hu Tang and Mu Fang Ji Tang pattern

FORMULA: Chai Hu 10g, Huang Qin 10g, Zhi Shi 15g, Ban Xia 10g, Bai Shao 15g, Da Zao 3 pieces, Sheng Jiang 5 slices, Han Fang Ji 10g, Shi Gao 60g, Gui Zhi 10g, Dang Shen 15g. (Ten packets, one packet per day. After taking five packets, pause for one day.)

SECOND VISIT: November 8th, 2015

After taking the herbs, the patient's chest oppression and occipital head pain were reduced, and his infraorbital and lower leg edema completely resolved. He averaged two bowel movements per day, each with a larger volume of stool, and his urine volume per trip increased while total trips per day and night decreased. However, the patient's full-body tremors, insomnia, leg weakness, substernal hard glomus, and gallbladder knocking pain did not noticeably improve, so I continued with the following formula:

Chaihu 10g, Huangqin 10g, Zhi Shi 10g, Ban Xia 10g, Bai Shao 15g, Da Zao 3 pieces, Sheng Jiang 5 slices, Han Fang Ji 10g, Shi Gao 60g, Gui Zhi 10g, Dang Shen 15g. (Ten packets, pause one day after taking 5 packets)

THIRD VISIT: November 22nd, 2015

After two weeks of taking herbs, the full-body tremors, insomnia, and leg weakness noticeably improved and the patient reported a strong recovery of his overall condition. However, the patient still had fullness and

---

[5] The substernal hard glomus corresponds to a Mu Fang Ji Tang pattern. Typically, the sub-sternum should be quite hard to the touch and the abdomen should feel full.

discomfort in the chest and rib-side, substernal hard glomus, and gall-bladder knocking pain. I continued with the previous formula:

Chaihu 10g, Huangqin 10g, Zhi Shi 10g, Ban Xia 10g, Bai Shao 15g, Da Zao 3 pieces, Sheng Jiang 5 slices, Han Fang Ji 10g, Shi Gao 60g, Gui Zhi 10g, Dang Shen 15g. (Ten packets, pause one day after taking five packets)

CLINICAL INSIGHT

At the time of writing, the patient's condition is stable, but the persistence of his abnormal abdominal presentation suggests that he might experience a relapse in the future.

Given the complex nature of this case, it would likely be difficult to establish a clear formula pattern without the guidance of abdominal palpation. As Yumoto Kyūshin noted in his essay, "The Importance of Abdominal Presentations and Abdominal Palpation Diagnosis" from *Imperial Han Medicine* (皇漢醫學): "The abdomen is the source of life itself and is thus at the root of all disease. As such, abdominal palpation is an indispensable aspect of diagnosis."

In Mu Fang Ji Tang, it is actually best to use Han Fang Ji. This is based upon the clinical experience of Keisetsu Ōtsuka (大塚敬節) and is worth noting.

Cerebral Stroke Sequelae Treated with
Gui Zhi Tang plus Fu Zi, Bai Zhu, Fu Ling

---

70 YEARS, MALE

HISTORY: The patient has a history of hypertension for twenty years and takes anti-hypertensive medication daily. Two months ago, he suddenly fell and lost consciousness. Further examination at a local hospital revealed he had suffered a cerebral ischemic stroke. After treatment, his condition improved and he was released from the hospital, but he still suffered from complete paralysis of his right arm and leg.

FIRST VISIT: April 17th, 2006

CURRENT: The patient has an average or slightly thin build, appears fatigued and weak, and current blood pressure is normal. He displays right-side paralysis, is unable to walk, has weak handgrip strength and retains some limited mobility in his right leg. The patient reports aversion to cold and wind, cold limbs, spontaneous sweating, weak urine stream, and occasional leg edema. He reports having good sleep and normal bowel movements.

TONGUE: Engorged, pale and dark with a thin white coating

PULSE: Moderate

ABDOMINAL PALPATION: Weak abdominal muscles and palpitations felt at the navel.

The patient was unwilling to receive acupuncture, so I first tried Gui Zhi Tang plus Fu Zi, Bai Zhu, Fu Ling.

FORMULA: Gui Zhi 10g, Bai Shao 10g, Gan Cao 5g, Sheng Jiang 5 slices, Da Zao 3 pieces, Fu Zi 10g, Bai Zhu 10g, Fu Ling 15g.

After one month of taking this formula, the patient's condition noticeably improved: his grip strength increased, and he was able to walk around his house using crutches. I continued to prescribe this formula with various modifications for six months, after which the patient was able to walk slowly without crutches and eat using chopsticks. He was able to perform most daily tasks, and his overall condition remained stable.

CLINICAL INSIGHT

Despite having hypertension for twenty years, the patient had avoided hemorrhagic stroke through successful regulation of his blood pressure with antihypertensive medication. Yet, despite these efforts, he still ended up suffering an ischemic stroke. Thus, people ought to consider the advantages and disadvantages of using western medical antihypertensive medication.

Jīngfāng herbalism can be effective in preventing strokes and treating their sequelae. Based upon analysis of a large number of stroke cases I have treated using the jīngfāng formula pattern identification method, I have found that most replete cases display Da Chai Hu Tang, San Huang Xie Xin Tang, Chai Hu Jia Long Gu Mu Li Tang, or Fang Feng Tong Sheng San patterns, while vacuity cases typically present with Jin Gui Shen Qi Wan, Zhen Gan Xi Feng Tang, or Bu Yang Huan Wu Tang patterns. Patients without clear replete or vacuity proclivities often respond to Gui Zhi Tang Jia Fu Zi, Bai Zhu, Fu Ling or Xiao Xu Ming Tang. Among those patients, overweight patients more often tend to present with Xiao Xu

Ming Tang patterns in stroke sequelae, while skinny patients more often tend to present with Gui Zhi Tang Jia Fu Zi, Bai Zhu, Fu Ling patterns.

Gui Zhi Tang Jia Fu Zi, Bai Zhu, Fu Ling is really just Gui Zhi Tang combined with Ling Gui Zhu Gan Tang and Zhen Wu Tang. Professor Liu Du-zhou (劉渡舟) believes that water qi counterflow is a common mechanism in ischemic stroke and, indeed, Ling Gui Zhu Gan Tang and Zhen Wu Tang are the two primary formulas for the treatment of water qi. Ostensibly, there are deeper layers of meaning beneath pattern formula correspondence worthy of further investigation.

The jīngfāng school has a very different understanding of the approach to diagnosis and treatment of stroke than most post-classical commentators. Theoretical discourse regarding "true wind strike" and "wind-like strike" which focuses too much on mechanisms and pathogenesis of disease is not that consistent with actual clinical reality. The misguided teachings of our forebears lead new students of Chinese medicine astray and made them scared to use warm, acrid formulas to treat stroke. In, *On Wind-Strike: Commentary and Criticism* (中風斠詮), the Republican era physician Zhang Shan-lei (張山雷) expressed extreme opposition to the use of Xu Ming Tang and other warm, acrid formulas in the treatment of stroke and said of Chen Xiu-yuan (陳修園) and Yu Jia-yan (喻嘉言), who were earlier proponents of the formula, "their theories might be new and interesting, but their patients surely all died."

Don't use the conclusions of modern pharmacology as a gold standard in your practice of pattern identification. In modern times, the use of Ma Huang and Gui Zhi in patients with hypertension and stroke is often prohibited due to the fact that these herbs can elevate blood pressure. Indeed, the label on most granule bottles for the formula Fang Feng Tong Sheng San, a formula that is extremely effective at preventing stroke, cautions against using the formula in stroke and hypertension for this very reason. In actuality, the efficacy of Fang Feng Tong Sheng San, Gui Zhi Tang Jia Bai Zhu, Fu Ling, Fu Zi, and Xu Ming Tang in stroke sequelae has been born out through extensive clinical experimentation, not subjective reasoning and theory crafting. In the Tang Dynasty, the sequelae of stroke were primarily treated with Gui Zhi Tang Jia Bai Zhu,

Fu Ling, Fu Zi, Xu Ming Tang, and other similar formulas. In *Essential Formulas Worth a Thousand in Gold*(千金要方, qiānjīn yàofāng), there are 10 different formulas with the name Xu Ming Tang (續命湯, extending life decoction) including four versions of Da Xu Ming Tang, Xiao Xu Ming Tang, Ma Huang Xu Ming Tang, Xu Ming Zhu San, and Xi Zhou Xu Ming Tang among others. These formulas, which are all implicated in the treatment of stroke, all use warm, acrid herbs and play an active role in improving cardiovascular and neurovascular circulation. In Japan, there was a famous case in which the 16th century physician Gensaku Manase (曲直瀨玄朔) treated and cured the then emperor's stroke using Xu Ming Tang. If Manase wasn't supremely confident in his diagnosis and treatment, he certainly wouldn't dare use a formula like Xu Ming Tang on the emperor.

Serum pharmacology and serum pharmacochemistry is a new direction in research that should be taken seriously. In serum pharmacology, pharmacological experiments and analysis are conducted not on herbal compounds, but on a serum extract taken from a lab animal that has been fed the herbal compound. Obtaining a serum extract from a lab animal that has digested, distributed, metabolized, and excreted elements of an herbal compound represents a truer picture of the actual pharmacological mechanisms possibly induced by the herb in the in vivo environment of the body. This form of research is particularly suitable for evaluating the efficacy of and ascertaining the pharmacomechanisms of herbs and formulas. Serum pharmacochemistry and pharmacodynamics research may also be useful for these purposes.

Serum pharmacochemistry primarily studies molecular compounds within serum and analyzes the effects and patterns of metabolism in externally absorbed active compounds. It is a rapidly developing and relatively accurate method of researching the material basis of Chinese herbal medicinals' mechanisms of action.

Serum pharmacochemistry presents the following advantages (over conventional methods of research): 1.) Prevents the possible skewing of experimental results due to physical properties of the prepared herbal compounds (varying pH values or osmotic properties of electrolytes, tannins etc.) and can simulate the in vivo state of the herb while still exploiting the advantages of an in vitro methodology. 2.) Helps avoid some of the erroneous conclusions reached by pure in vitro experiments.

That said, serum pharmacochemistry research also has its disadvantages: 1.) After being absorbed in the GI tract, some active compounds of Chinese medicinals will appear in plasma preparations as opposed to serum preparations. 2.) In the process of separating the serum from the blood through blood clotting, a series of enzymes are activated, and lysosomes are released, these enzymes and lysosomes may denature certain medicinal compounds. 3.) Serum processing and inactivation might lead to a loss of materials released by medicinals or medicinal vectors. As such, serum pharmacochemistry has limited application in the research of thrombi and coagulation. Serum pharmacochemistry is primarily applicable to research regarding Chinese medicinals that exert their effect after absorption into the blood. This method is less useful for researching topical medicine, targeted drug delivery, and medicinals that work by directly stimulating the GI tract.

With the advent of serum pharmacochemistry research, a new era in Chinese medical formula research has arrived. This new form of research provides the technology to understand and elucidate the material basis of Chinese medicinals' efficacy and mechanisms. The combination of serum pharmacochemistry and serum pharmacology will indeed be helpful in unlocking the secret to the material basis of the effects that Chinese medicinals exert on the body. Additionally, Chinese medicine chemical fingerprinting has emerged as a new model and system for basic research on Chinese herbs. If Chinese medicine chemical fingerprinting can be combined with serum pharmacochemistry, these two new technologies will help produce an even clearer picture of the material basis of Chinese herbal pharmacological mechanisms.

Chronic Gastritis Treated with Xiang Su Yin

AGE UNDISCLOSED, FEMALE

Patient complains of stomach distention, frequent burping, and chest oppression among other symptoms. She was diagnosed with chronic superficial gastritis by a western medical hospital. She reports that she has always had "stomach cold" and will produce copious saliva after eating any "cold" food. Aside from these symptoms, the patient's symptom and abdominal palpation presentation were otherwise unremarkable. Upon palpating the spine, the patient reported pain with pressure below the seventh thoracic spinous process at DU9.

Based upon the above symptoms, I prescribed 3 packets of Xiang Su Yin.

FORMULA: Xiang Fu 10g, Su Geng 10g, Chen Pi 10g, Gan Cao 3g, Gao Liang Jiang 3g, Da Zao 3 pieces. Additionally, I advised the patient to lie on a heating pad or hot compress centered at DU9 before sleep each night. I explained that this would help reinforce treatment efficacy.

After taking the medicine for just three days, the patient called me and excitedly informed me that the herbs had been very effective: her stomach distention, burping, and chest oppression had noticeably subsided. After taking just five packets, all her symptoms resolved. In clinical practice I like combining jīngfāng formula pattern identification treatment with acupuncture, bloodletting, massage, and other modalities — I find this combination to be particularly effective.

Frequent Nausea, Lack of Appetite and other Gastrointestinal Symptoms Treated with Da Chai Hu Tang plus San Huang Xie Xin Tang

MIDDLE-AGED, FEMALE

The patient has a strong build, a ruddy complexion, and lists several GI related complaints that have gotten worse in the past half year. A battery of western medical tests ruled out cancer or any tumor-related pathology, but treatment had thus far been ineffective. She had also been to several Chinese doctors, including some very respectable ones, but none had resolved her condition.

I asked my daughter, who is also a doctor, to treat this patient, but the patient seemed a bit hesitant because my daughter was relatively inexperienced. On the basis of the patient's chest and rib-side fullness and discomfort, substernal pain upon pressing, bitter taste in the mouth, nausea and vomiting, poor appetite, constipation, yellow urine, red tongue with yellow coating, and strong build, etc., she prescribed a combination of Da Chai Hu Tang and San Huang Xie Xin Tang.

After reviewing the patient's case, I thought the formula corresponded well with the presentation, so I signed off on her prescription. After six days, the patient excitedly returned to our clinic and reported that her symptoms all noticeably subsided after the first dose and after five, all symptoms resolved. However, upon palpating her abdomen, I found that the patient still had some substernal pain upon pressure, so I made a few slight modifications to the existing formula. Only after another month of herbs did the patient's substernal pain upon pressure fully resolve.

Later on, the patient returned to our clinic complaining of a relapse in symptoms due to overeating during the holidays combined with catching a cold. Again, I gave the case to my daughter, but this time the patient's attitude was one of upmost confidence, a far cry from when she came for her first visit.

CLINICAL INSIGHT

This case demonstrates the simplicity and practicality of formula pattern diagnosis and highlights the invaluable nature of abdominal palpation and abdominal presentations, facets of diagnosis strongly emphasized by Zhang Zhong-jing himself. Unfortunately, after the Tang dynasty, practice and study of jīngfāng slowly declined and abdominal palpation diagnosis was all but forgotten. After Tōdō Yoshimasu (吉益東洞) proclaimed, "the symptom pattern should be prioritized over pulse and abdominal presentation should be prioritized over pattern", there was a resurgence of interest in abdominal diagnosis among *kampo* practitioners. Yet, strangely, the renewed enthusiasm for the study and use of abdominal diagnosis never spread to China. How would we have known about the patient's chest and rib-side fullness and discomfort and substernal pain upon pressing if not through abdominal palpation? This is why previous doctors who treated the patient failed to grasp her pattern with formulas like Ban Xia Xie Xin Tang, Huang Qi Jian Zhong Tang, and Xiang Su Yin.

Whenever we palpate a classic abdominal presentation, it increases the accuracy of our formula pattern diagnosis and substantially increases our chances of successfully treating the patient's illness. In my many decades of practice, I have always incorporated abdominal palpation into my diagnosis and the abdominal presentation has become the most important factor in my identification of formula patterns. It gives me an empty feeling and unsettles me to see doctors not using abdominal diagnosis in their treatment. I just don't understand why someone wouldn't avail themselves of such a useful form of diagnosis!?

Atrophic Gastritis with Mid-Grade Intestinal Metaplasia Treated with Gui Zhi Xin Jia Tang (Tàiyáng-Tàiyīn Combination Disease Type)

Ms. Hu, 40 years

FIRST VISIT: October 5th, 1996

The patient has suffered from gastrointestinal issues for years and was diagnosed with atrophic gastritis and intestinal metaplasia via endoscopy. The patient reports that for six months, she's had dull pain in her stomach which is lessened with massage, depressed mood, significant weight loss, frequent night sweating, nasal congestion with rhinorrhea, occasional feverish sensation with agitation, poor appetite, dry heaving in the morning, loose, thin stools, light sleep, frequent dreams from which she is scared awake, scant menses and delayed onset, and heaviness, weakness, and soreness of her joints. She has a slightly diminutive and thin build and a sickly, white pallor. Additionally, she reports being averse to wind with limbs that easily feel cold, averse to heat in the summer with copious sweating, and gets colds easily in the fall and winter.

TONGUE: Thick white coating

PULSE: Floating, moderate, and forceless

ABDOMINAL PALPATION: Flat stomach with tight abdominal muscles, hard substernal glomus with slight pain upon pressing.

DIAGNOSIS: Tàiyáng disease with vacuous defense yáng leading to invasion of cold-damp into tàiyīn, ultimately resulting in dysfunctional upbearing and downbearing of the spleen and stomach. Thus, the treatment strategy should be to harmonize defense and construction, supplement qi, and moderate the stomach.

FORMULA: Gui Zhi Xin Jia Tang: Gui Zhi 15g, Bai Shao 15g, Dang Shen 15g, Zhi Gan Cao 5g, Da Zao 3 pieces, Sheng Jiang 5 slices. (Five packets)

After taking the herbs, the patient felt a bit more comfortable and reported a lessening of aversion to wind and rhinorrhea. After taking another fifteen packets, the patient reported significant reduction in stomach pain and night sweats, her stools had become more formed, and the thick tongue coating had receded. The formula clearly matched the patient's pattern, so I continued to use this formula for another three months with modifications while also using stick moxa on RN13, RN12, and DU9 among other points. At the end of the three months, the patient's symptoms completely resolved. After discontinuing herbal treatment, I advised the patient to continue moxaing RN12, RN6, RN4, and ST36 among other points to reinforce the effects of treatment. On May 16th, 1997, endoscopy revealed that the atrophic gastritis and intestinal metaplasia had resolved, and only superficial gastritis remained.

In a follow-up five years later, the patient reported they had never experienced a relapse of symptoms.

CLINICAL INSIGHT

I used Gui Zhi Xin Jia Tang in this case for the following four reasons: 1.) The *Treatise on Cold Damage* states: "After inducing sweating and there is body pain and a sunken, slow pulse.... Xin Jia Tang is indicated." The "floating pulse" in this case does not conform to this description, but the mechanism and cause of disease are consistent with the Xin Jia Tang formula pattern. 2.) The patient had many signs of a "Gui Zhi constitution."

She had a thin build, a pallid complexion, expressive eyes, tendency to sweat, recurrent cold, and a flat abdomen with tight abdominal muscles. 3.) The clinical presentation in this case was consistent with a Gui Zhi Tang pattern: Aversion to wind, feeling of heat and agitation, sweating, nasal congestion, heaving, and a floating, moderate pulse. 4.) Yumoto Kyūshin noted: "The use of Ren Shen is indicated in weakness of the stomach with hard glomus due to a decline in metabolic function." (In the Han dynasty, when Zhang Zhong-jing was practicing, Ren Shen referred to Dang Shen.) This patient presented with spleen vacuity and a substernal hard glomus abdominal presentation, so I selected Gui Zhi Xin Jia Tang, which contains Ren Shen.

Chronic Atrophic Gastritis Treated with a Combination of Xiao Chai Hu Tang, Xiao Xian Xiong Tang and Ling Gui Zhu Gan Tang (Shàoyáng Disease type)

Ms. Bao, 42 years

First visit: November 15th, 1997

The patient has suffered from stomach pain for years and was diagnosed with severe chronic atrophic gastritis and high-grade intestinal meta-plasia three years ago. The patient reports that for the past six months she has suffered from continuous weight loss, headache, tightness in the nape of the neck with restricted movement upon turning or raising the head, and periocular edema in the morning. In terms of digestive symptoms, the patient reports pain and distention in the stomach which is triggered by eating and is less when hungry, gassy distention in the stomach that fails to result in belching, and frequent vomiting of bit-ter, turbid bolus which slightly relieves GI symptoms. Additionally, the patient complains of constipation (one BM every four to five days), exac-erbation of symptoms when upset emotionally, swollen gums and canker sores that often accompany onset of stomach pain and make chewing painful, poor appetite, copious salty saliva, and copious leukorrhea.

Tongue: Dark and pale red with a greasy, moist, yellow coating

Pulse: Sunken and wiry

ABDOMINAL PALPATION: Substernal distention, fullness and palpitation, water splash sound upon tapping, and pain upon pressing. Rib-side discomfort and right-side dull knocking pain that radiates to below the sternum.

This case has a complicated symptom presentation, but from a disease mechanism perspective, this is clearly a case of shàoyáng qì stagnation, phlegm-heat bind, and water-rheum counterflow. As such, the method of treatment is to course the shàoyáng qì dynamic, clear and transform phlegm-heat, disinhibit water, and descend counterflow. To accomplish this, I used a combination of Xiao Chai Hu Tang, Xiao Xian Xiong Tang, and Ling Gui Zhu Gan Tang: Chai Hu 10g, Gui Zhi 10g, Bai Shao 10g, Bai Zhu 10g, Ban Xia 10g, Quan Gua Lou 15g, Fu Ling 15g, Sheng Jiang 5 slices, Huang Lian 5g (Five packets)

SECOND VISIT: The patient reported that after taking the third packet, they began feeling gurgling in their stomach, frequently burped and passed gas, and noticed significantly more disinhibited urine and bowel movements. After five packets, the canker sores and swollen gums resolved and the substernal dull pain reduced by half, however the neck tightness remained. This reaction was reminiscent of a description of "qì phase disease" in the *Essential Prescriptions of the Golden Cabinet*: "When yīn and yáng are brought into connection, qì moves freely. As the great qì turns, its qì disperses. In replete cases, this results in the passing of gas, in vacuity cases it leads to urinary incontinence." Clearly, the formula was a good match for this disease presentation, so I prescribed another five packets and used a bone-rightening manipulation to correct deviations at the third and fourth cervical spinous processes.

THIRD VISIT: The patient's stomach pain had basically completely subsided and her only remaining complaints were occasional abdominal distention and lack of appetite. These symptoms were indications of the qì dynamic still not being completely regulated and coursed, so I used Liu Jun Zi Tang to address the remaining issues. After continuing to use various modifications of Liu Jun Zi Tang for another two months and advising the patient to massage LI4 when they had time, all the patient's symptoms subsided. Subsequent endoscopy revealed that the atrophic gastritis and intestinal metaplasia had disappeared, leaving only some mild superficial gastritis. In a follow-up three years later, the patient reported there had been no relapse of symptoms.

CLINICAL INSIGHT

Xiao Chai Hu Tang is the primary formula in the treatment of shàoyáng disease. In the modifications for the formula it states, "If there is abdominal pain, remove Huang Qin and add Shao Yao" and "If there is substernal palpitation and inhibited urine, remove Huang Qin and add Fu Ling." I achieved success in this case by strictly following these modifications through multiple visits.

The *Treatise on Cold Damage* attaches particular importance to abdominal diagnosis. For instance, Zhang Zhong-jing describes abdominal presentations for all three of the formulas used in the prescription above: For Xiao Chai Hu Tang he gives, "chest and rib-side discomfort and fullness" and "hard glomus below the ribs", for Xiao Xian Xiong Tang he gives, "pain upon pressing below the sternum" and for Ling Gui Zhu Gan Tang, "substernal counterflow fullness", "substernal palpitations" and "substernal water splash sound on tapping." The objective nature of abdominal presentations makes them easy to grasp. In this case, I easily identified the targets of treatment by identifying and matching these abdominal presentations.

The *Treatise on Cold Damage* states: "In chest bind, there can also be tightness of the neck similar to the presentation in soft tetany." Clearly, there is an internal connection between neck tightness and chest bind or stomach pain. In my own clinical practice, I've found that if chest bind is accompanied by cervical spinous process subluxations that induce neck tightness and pain, correcting the subluxations can resolve the chest bind, so the use of cervical manipulations in the swift treatment of this disease cannot be underestimated.

Moderate Atrophic Gastritis Treated with a Combination of Zhi Zi Chi Tang, Ban Xia Hou Pu Tang and Xiao Chai Hu Tang (Yángmíng-Shàoyáng Combination Disease Type)

MR. LIN, 40 YEARS

FIRST VISIT: March 9th, 1999

HISTORY: For ten years, the patient has suffered from fullness and glomus of the substernal stomach area that worsens after eating and he has become averse to eating as a result. During this time, his bowel movements have alternated between constipation and sloppy stool and are often accompanied by tenesmus. After several endoscopies and biopsies, the patient was diagnosed with moderate atrophic gastritis of the antrum, gastric mucosal gland atrophy, and mid-grade intestinal metaplasia.

CURRENT: The patient has a large build and a dark, sallow complexion. He complains of glomus and distention below the sternum, clamoring stomach which is worse at night, chest oppression, and flusteredness and agitation that make it difficult to get to sleep. Additionally, the patient reports having a bitter taste in the mouth and dryness in the throat upon waking, and expectorating sticky, pale yellow phlegm. He often feels nauseous, reports feeling a plum-pit sensation in his throat and has scant, dark urine.

TONGUE: Dark, pale red with a thick, greasy, yellow coating.

ABDOMINAL PALPATION: Fullness and distention in the chest and below the sternum with an intensification of oppression in the chest upon pressing. The upper abdomen is soft and there is no pain upon pressing, but there is dull knocking pain in the lower right rib-side and discomfort upon pressing below the left and right ribcage.

DIAGNOSIS: This is a case of shàoyáng qì dynamic breakdown with damp, turbid phlegm and heat stagnating in yángmíng. As such, the treatment should aim to clear heat, eliminate vexation, undo binds, transform phlegm, course qi, and descend counterflow. To execute this treatment strategy, I prescribed a combination of Zhi Zi Chi Tang, Ban Xia Hou Pu Tang, and Xiao Chai Hu Tang: Zhi Zi 10g, Dou Chi 10g, Huang Qin 10g, Ban Xia 10g, Su Geng 10g, Fu Ling 10g, Chai Hu 6g, Hou Pu 6g, Sheng Jiang 3 slices. (Five packets)

After taking the first five packets, the results were unremarkable, but there were also no adverse reactions. After another five packets, there was gradual improvement. There was a significant improvement in distention after eating, bowel movements were regular, the tongue coating began to thin, and the stomach clamoring and other symptoms began to gradually subside. Given the noticeable improvement in symptoms, I prescribed another seven packets, this time removing Huang Qin.

Most symptoms gradually subsided and the yellow, greasy coating continued to recede, but the patient still complained of plum-pit qì in the throat and occasional chest oppression. I gave seven packets of the original formula but decreased the doses proportionally and added 6g each of Xuan Fu Hua, Quan Gua Lou, and Yu Jin to further coarse and clear. After those seven packets, the patient's condition was already significantly resolved. After that, I used a modification of Chai Shao Liu Jun Zi Tang to continue reinforcing and recuperating the patient's condition. Additionally, I advised the patient to massage DU9, ST36, and PC6 among other points. After another two months of treatment, the patient's condition completely resolved. On July 20th, 1999, a further endoscopy found the atrophic gastritis had healed and only superficial gastritis remained. In a follow-up two years later, the patient reported that besides the occasional discomfort after overeating or drinking alcohol, he hadn't experienced any discomfort since.

CLINICAL INSIGHT

Atrophic gastritis is often accompanied by "stomach clamoring". In Chinese medicine, "stomach clamoring" refers to a rather difficult to describe feeling of hunger and pain without actually being hungry or in pain and a sense of vexation and vacuity agitation. This presentation corresponds quite closely to the symptom presentation in the Zhi Zi Chi Tang pattern: "Vacuity agitation with inability to sleep that can progress to vexation and restlessness" and "a hot and agitated feeling with chest oppression". This patient presented with substernal glomus and fullness, stomach clamoring, vexation, chest oppression, flusteredness, agitation and insomnia, and scant, dark urine - a presentation that corresponds to the Zhi Zi Chi Tang pattern. Additionally, the plum-pit qì and copious thick phlegm suggested a phlegm-qi binding mechanism typical of a Ban Xia Hou Pu Tang pattern, as well as bitter taste in the mouth, throat dryness, and rib-side discomfort and fullness which suggest a breakdown of the shàoyáng qì dynamic found in the Xiao Chai Hu Tang pattern. As such, these three formulas were combined with good results.

Atrophic Gastritis with Compound Ulcer Treated with Modified Huang Qi Jian Zhong Tang

MR. PAN, 45 YEARS

FIRST VISIT: October 12, 1998.

The patient has suffered from stomach pain that has gradually worsened over the last twelve years. In the past three years, he continually lost weight, suffered from fatigue, and was eventually diagnosed with atrophic gastritis, compound ulcer, and intestinal metaplasia via endoscopy and other tests.

The illness took a deep emotional toll on the patient, and this was reflected in his emaciated build, haggard appearance, sallow complexion, and look of desolation in his eyes. He complained of profuse sweating, a feeling of heaviness in the body, weakness of his muscles, a bitter taste in the mouth, dry throat, agitated heat in the hands and feet, and periorbital edema upon waking. He also complained of stomach pain that lessened with heat and massage and worsened when hungry. His appetite was poor, his stomach distended, and bowel movements dry, infrequent (one every three to four days) and at times bloody. Finally, he also complained of insomnia, frequent startled wakeups, nocturnal emissions, and heavy night sweats that would soak through his shirt.

PULSE: Thin and forceless

TONGUE: Engorged, pale red with a thin white coating.

ABDOMINAL PALPATION: A flat and slightly concave abdomen with tight, rigid abdominal muscles. Strong palpitations felt at either side of the navel.

DIAGNOSIS: Spleen yáng vacuity Tàiyīn disease. The treatment should warm the middle, supplement qì, nourish blood, and clear heat.

FORMULA: Modified Huang Qi Jian Zhong Tang: Gui Zhi 15g, Dang Gui 15g, Pu Gong Ying 15g, Zhi Huang Qi 30g, Chao Bai Shao 30g, Yi Tang 30g, Gao Liang Jiang 3g, Da Zao 5 pieces, Chuan Lian Zi 10g, Yan Hu Suo 10g, Zhi Gan Cao 10g. (Seven packets)

SECOND VISIT: The patient reported that after taking the herbs, he could feel warmth circulating in his stomach, after which his bowel movements became regular, the pain in his stomach was reduced, and he felt relaxed and sleepy. After taking the same formula with various modifications for two months, his hunger-induced stomach pain subsided and only mildly relapsed if he overate, became overly emotional, or the weather became too cold or rainy. These were signs that the chronic stomach illness had already entered the collaterals, so I added San Qi 3g and Wei Pi (Hedgehog hide) 6g. I continued to modify the formula to fit his pattern over the course of another three months. During this time, I advised him to not overeat and to refrain from anger and agitation. Gradually, his strength and energy recovered, and at the end of those three months the stomach pain had completely resolved.

Six months later, an endoscopy showed that the patient's atrophic gastritis, intestinal metaplasia, and compound ulcer had all healed, leaving only superficial gastritis. Upon a follow up two years later, the patient reported he hadn't had any relapse of pain since.

Clinical Insight

The formula pattern for Xiao Jian Zhong Tang in Tàiyīn disease is, "Urgent pain in the abdomen", "palpitations and agitation" and "taxation with interior urgency, palpitations, nose bleeding, pain in the abdomen, nocturnal emissions, weakness of the four limbs, agitation and heat in the hands and feet, and dryness of the mouth and throat." The patient's interior heat-related symptoms such as the "palpitations, insomnia, constipation, bloody stools, nocturnal emissions, night sweats, agitation and heat of the hands and feet, and dry mouth and throat" are all due to what Li Dong-yuan (李東垣) calls "yīn fire rising and overtaking earth."

As such, it is clear that Zhang Zhong-jing's Xiao Jian Zhong Tang paved the way for the "treating heat with warm-sweet medicinals" method popularized in the post-classical period. In this case, I didn't approach the heat symptoms using the common yin-nourishing method found today, instead opting to treat the presentation as a Tàiyīn disease and using a modified Xiao Jian Zhong Tang.

I decided to add Huang Qi for the following reasons: 1.) The patient had a "Huang Qi constitution", evidenced by his gaunt and haggard facial appearance, sallow complexion, lack of animation in his eyes, weak muscles, and engorged, pale tongue. 2.) Apart from presenting with typical symptoms of a Xiao Jian Zhong Tang pattern, the patient also had the "vacuity" symptoms and signs described in the *Golden Cabinet* taxation disease section. For instance, he had spontaneous sweating, night sweats, periorbital edema, and heaviness of the body, among other symptoms. Indeed, "sweating with edema" is an archetypal "Huang Qi pattern" presentation.

Superficial Atrophic Gastritis with Mid-Grade Intestinal Metaplasia Treated with Huang Lian E Jiao Tang plus Mai Men Dong Tang (Shàoyīn Disease Type)

MR. XU, 40 YEARS

FIRST VISIT: September 20th, 1999

HISTORY: The patient has a weak constitution and a history of hypertension and dull stomach pain of a burning, roaming nature accompanied by agitation, feeling of hunger with no desire to eat, lack of satisfaction from food, and stomach clamoring. He was diagnosed with superficial atrophic gastritis, intestinal metaplasia, and hypochlorhydria via endoscopy. He had taken Mai Dong, Sha Shen, Mu Gua, and Sheng Di for years with little benefit.

CURRENT: The patient has a gaunt build, flushed red cheeks, complains of vexing heat in the five hearts, insomnia, night sweats, dry mouth, bitter taste in the mouth, frequent eructation, palpitations, and scant, yellow urine. The patient reports that the pain is worse when hungry and is accompanied by a burning sensation, clamoring, and vexation which makes it difficult to fall asleep.

PULSE: Wiry, thin, and rapid

TONGUE: Tender, red tongue with very thin coating

ABDOMINAL PALPATION: The abdomen is flat, and the abdominal muscles are paper-thin and insubstantial. He reports a subjective feeling of distention and glomus in the sub-sternum and upon pressing, there is hard glomus that gives way on deeper pressure and completely lacks spring.

DIAGNOSIS: This presentation is characteristic of the yīn vacuity and dry heat in shàoyīn transforming to heat syndrome. Treatment should focus on nourishing yīn, draining heat, and using acridity to unblock and relieve pain.

FORMULA: A combination of Huang Lian E Jiao Tang and Mai Men Dong Tang: Mai Dong 20g, E Jiao 10g, Sheng Bai Shao 10g, Huang Lian 3g, Sheng Gan Cao 3g, Huang Qin 3g, Ban Xia 3g, Jing Mi (handful). (Five packets)

After taking the herbs, there was no notable change in symptoms, but no adverse reactions either. Given that the formula matched the pattern well, I didn't make any changes and prescribed another seven packets. After the second week of herbs, the patient's burning sensation in the stomach decreased, so I stuck with the same formula but switched out Huang Qin for Zhi Zi 6g, Pu Gong Ying 15g.

After finishing the above round of herbs, the patient reported better sleep, improved appetite, and reduction in stomach pain. However, he still complained of stomach clamoring. I knew that I had arrived at the right formula, so I continued prescribing it with various modifications and after eighty days, all symptoms resolved. On a follow-up two years later, the patient had gained weight and said he never had any relapse in pain symptoms.

CLINICAL INSIGHT

The Emergency Standby Remedies (肘後備急方) states that Huang Lian E Jiao Tang is indicated for "Vacuity vexation, insomnia, and anxious brooding in the aftermath of a serious illness." *Kampo* physician Yōdō Odai (尾台榕堂) offered this incisive analysis: "(Huang Lian E Jiao Tang) and Zhi Zi Chi Tang have similar symptom presentations but varying pathomechanisms." In my clinical experience, both formula patterns present with stomach clamoring, burning pain, anxious brooding and vexing heat, insomnia, and palpitations. The difference between the two is that Huang Lian E Jiao Tang is a shàoyīn transforming to heat yīn vacuity internal heat syndrome, whereas Zhi Zi Chi Tang is a yángmíng disease with lingering evil heat syndrome. The main difference between these otherwise similar presentations is one of vacuity and repletion.

Mai Men Dong Tang uses sweet, cool herbs that moisten to treat yin and fluid vacuity with concomitant qì counterflow of the lung and stomach, but pain is often due to congestion which can only be remedied with acrid herbs; therefore, Mai Men Dong Tang also includes Ban Xia in a 1:7 ration with Mai Men Dong. This combination of an acrid herb to unblock and descend counterflow combined with a large dose of sweet, cool, moistening herbs ensures that the cool moistening won't lead to stagnation and the acrid opening won't cause dryness.

Moderate Atrophic Gastritis with Intestinal Metaplasia Treated with Wu Zhu Yu Tang plus Li Zhong Tang (Juéyīn-Tàiyīn combination Disease Type)

MS. WANG, 62 YEARS

FIRST VISIT: December 20ᵗʰ, 1999

HISTORY: The patient has suffered from stomach illness for twenty years. In recent years, she has had cold stomach pain nearly every day, counterflow of "cold qì", chest and rib-side counterflow and fullness, and dry heaving. She typically has two to three bowel movements per day with sloppy, thin stool. She was diagnosed with moderate atrophic gastritis and intestinal metaplasia via endoscopy and biopsy. She was diagnosed with chronic colitis via colonoscopy.

CURRENT: The patient has a gaunt, tall build, appears fatigued, and has a pallid and slightly sallow complexion. She complains of poor appetite, excessive saliva, frequent eructation, and occasional vomiting after ingesting food.

PULSE: Sunken and thin

TONGUE: Dark, pale red with a thick, moist, white coating.

ABDOMINAL PALPATION: There is a feeling of heavy pressure below the sternum and a slightly distended quality upon palpation. Tapping and pushing the stomach yields a water splash sound and her chest and rib-side display glomus, fullness, and aversion to touch.

DIAGNOSIS: This is Juéyīn disease turbid yīn counterflow, lack of effusion of chest yáng, spleen yáng transformation dysfunction, and rheum congesting in the stomach with qì counterflow. This pathomechanism should be treated by warming the liver and stomach, unblocking yáng, and descending counterflow.

FORMULA: Apply the concept of the combination of Wu Zhu Yu Tang and Li Zhong Tang: Dang Shen 20g, Wu Zhu Yu 10g, Bai Zhu 10g, Sheng Jiang 10 slices, Da Zao 10 pieces. (Five packets)

ACUPUNCTURE: PC6 (Both sides), ST36 (Both sides), LR3 (Both Sides), DU20 retained for 15 minutes.

After acupuncture, the patient reported a significant reduction in nausea. However, two hours after taking the first packet of herbs, she developed a bad headache, stomach pain, vertigo, vexing heat, borborygmus, and had several bouts of diarrhea. I reconsidered every aspect of the patient's presentation and my prescription and concluded that the diagnosis was correct, so I asked her to continue taking the formula. Subsequent doses did not produce the same mìnxuàn reaction and all her symptoms were significantly relieved. Seeing that the formula had been effective, I prescribed another five packets at a lower dose and advised her to massage the four points listed above to reinforce the healing effect.

After finishing that round of herbs, the patient reported the "cold qì" counterflow feeling had vanished, but she still complained of a bitter taste in the mouth, dry mouth, poor appetite, sloppy stools, periorbital edema in the morning, and scant, yellow, inhibited urine.

PULSE: Sunken and wiry

TONGUE: Thin yellow coating

ABDOMINAL PALPATION: Substernal palpitation, water splash sound upon tapping, and a knotted feeling in the stomach.

DIAGNOSIS: The tàiyīn component of the disease was still present, but the Juéyīn aspect had pivoted out from yīn to yáng to become a shàoyáng disease. Treatment should focus on harmonizing and resolving shàoyáng, warming the middle, and transforming turbidity.

FORMULA: Modified Chaihu Guizhi Ganjiang Tang (Five packets.) Chai Hu 10g, Gui Zhi 10g, Tian Hua Fen 10g, Mu Li 10g, Fu Ling 10g, Bai Zhu 10g, Pu Gong Ying 10g, Gan Jiang 5g, Zhi Gan Cao 3g. (Five packets)

After taking the herbs, all symptoms were noticeably reduced and after taking sixty or so packets of various modifications of the above formula, all symptoms were resolved.

An endoscopy and biopsy performed on July 9th, 2000, confirmed that the previous stomach pathologies had all resolved. Upon follow-up one year later, I was overjoyed to see that the patient was still in good health.

CLINICAL INSIGHT

During the first visit, the patient experienced a mìnxuàn reaction after I prescribed her Wu Zhu Yu Tang on the basis of my diagnosis of juéyīn-tàiyīn combination disease with liver qì overwhelming the spleen and rheum counterflow. After continuing to use the same basic formula, her vomiting and nausea resolved, and her headache was significantly improved. At this time, there was shift in her pathology wherein "yáng recovered and yīn receded" and the Juéyīn disease shifted outward to shàoyáng disease. However, the patient's middle yáng had yet to recover, so the overall pathomechanism presented as a shàoyáng tàiyīn dragover disease.

The patient's main symptoms — chest and rib-side fullness with slight bind, inhibited urine, thirst but no vomiting, sweating only from the head, alternating heat effusion and aversion to cold, and agitation—corresponded precisely to the Chai Hu Gui Zhi Gan Jiang Tang pattern. However, due to the tendency toward brevity in the language of *The Treatise on Cold Damage*, the Chai Hu Gui Zhi Gan Jiang Tang line does not mention digestive symptoms like stomach pain, diarrhea, or abdominal distention. As such, it has been the task of later generations to expand upon the understanding and application of this formula pattern. In his *Analysis and Elaboration on "The Categorized Formulas"*, Yōdō Odai states: "(Chai Hu Gui Zhi Gan Jiang Tang) is indicated when there is sloppy stool, inhibited urine, pallid complexion, fatigue, and adverse response to stronger herbs." Liu Du-zhou comments that Chai Hu Gui Zhi Gan Jiang Tang "Functions like a combination of Xiao Chai Hu Tang and Li Zhong Tang." These later commentaries give us a clear understanding of the formula's function in digestive illness.

When treating Juéyīn disease, it is not a coincidence that these mìnxuàn reactions occur frequently, but is rather a sign of "yáng recovering and yīn receding". Yumoto Kyūshin has noted: "The statement in the *Classic of History* that 'In intractable diseases, there can be no cure without mìnxuàn' is an inviolable truth previously undiscovered by the ancients and has been wholeheartedly espoused by both physicians and patients." My own humble opinion is that the mìnxuàn reaction represents a destabilization of a "stable" pathological condition and a positive indication that the upright qi is recovering, and the illness is subsiding.

Atrophic Gastritis Treated with
Huang Qi Jian Zhong Tang plus Shen Qi Wan
(Spleen and Kidney Yang Deficiency Type)

MR. CAO, 30 YEARS

FIRST VISIT: May 3rd, 1997

HISTORY: The patient recalls being ill throughout his childhood and has a history of hepatitis. In recent years, he has suffered from cold pain in the stomach, stomach clamoring when hungry that is relieved with food, and occasional eructation. He was diagnosed with atrophic gastritis and Hepatitis B via endoscopy, biopsy, and Hepatitis B surface antigen testing.

CURRENT: Patient has a tall, gaunt build and appears fatigued. He complains of shortness of breath, spontaneous sweating, weakness of the lower back, aversion to cold and cold limbs, copious clear urine, and incomplete bowel movements with sloppy stool.

PULSE: Thin and moderate

TONGUE: Pale red with a thin white coating

ABDOMINAL PALPATION: Substernal pain upon pressing, but continued massage in the same area is comfortable. The abdominal muscles are thin, and the lower abdomen lacks springiness and gives out under pressure.

DIAGNOSIS: Spleen and Kidney dual yáng qì vacuity.

FORMULA: Huang Qi Jian Zhong Tang plus Shen Qi Wan (Seven packets)

After taking the herbs, the patient's appetite was marginally improved. I continued using the same formula for another month, after which all symptoms noticeably improved. After another two months using various modifications of this formula, symptoms continued to improve, the patient gained weight, his lower abdomen began to feel springier, and endoscopy revealed that the atrophic gastritis had receded.

However, the patient's urine became darker and malodorous, he was still HBsAg and Anti-HBs positive, and his SGPT had exceeded the normal range. I pivoted to Jin Gui Shen Qi Wan pills 10g twice daily, washed down with a decoction of Pu Gong Ying (30g) for forty-five days. However, an HBV-5 Panel Test revealed continued HBsAg and Anti-HBs positivity. I continued prescribing the same formula for another fifty days, after which a subsequent HBV-5 Panel Test revealed that the patient was now HBsAg positive and Anti-HBs negative. Additionally, his SGPT and SGOT had dropped within the normal range. After achieving this result, I suspended treatment and asked the patient to continue monitoring their condition. Three subsequent panel tests all yielded the same result, and the patient completely recovered.

CLINICAL INSIGHT

Atrophic gastritis and inactive carrier stage Hepatitis B are both considered chronic, intractable diseases. What makes these diseases so intractable is that the upright qì becomes weakened while evil toxins lodge deeply and congest the normal qì dynamic. As such, over time this stalemate between upright and evil qì progresses into a "stable" pathogenic dynamic. My approach to this type of chronic illness is as follows: 1.) Awaken the body's self-healing response to create an internal dynamic that begins to manifest clear symptoms of the pathology, 2.)

Strengthen the local feedback system to activate a physiological immune response, thereby shifting from an upright-evil stalemate condition to an activated response. 3.) Once symptoms start to appear, this signals that the organism's stable pathogenic dynamic is wavering and true healing from the illness can be achieved.

The most effective way to activate the immune system is to supplement and ensure the robustness of yáng qì. By shifting the stalemate between yáng qì and the evil toxic pathogen from a stable pathogenic dynamic to an activated, adversarial dynamic, the overall course of disease can be shortened. yáng qì is the source of the organism's warmth and Kidney yáng is the root of the whole body's yáng qì, thus it follows from this logic that Shen Qi Wan is an appropriate formula for this pathology. Indeed, using Shen Qi Wan is absolutely crucial for obtaining good results in these cases.

It is important to note that in the process of activating yáng qì, certain mìnxuàn symptoms and presentations like darker colored urine, high SGPT, etc., will invariably arise. However, this is to be expected and, as the *Classic of History* notes, "In intractable diseases, there can be no cure without a mìnxuàn reaction". As yáng qì continues to recover, the transient mìnxuàn symptoms will subside. To be safe, one can add one or two heat-clearing, toxin-resolving herbs to ease the symptoms.

Dumping Syndrome Subsequent to Stomach Surgery Treated with Xuan Fu Hua Tang

MALE, 67 YEARS

HISTORY: When the patient was 37 years old, he began experiencing stomach distention and frequent eructation after practicing qigong. One year later, he underwent gastrectomy but continued to suffer from distention and eructation even after the surgery. Subsequently, he was diagnosed with dumping syndrome by a local hospital. Because neither western nor Chinese medicine improved his condition, and his symptoms weren't particularly severe, he didn't continue to pursue treatment. However, in recent years, the distention and eructation worsened, and he also developed hypertension and coronary heart disease. One day last month, the patient's distention became extremely severe and radiated to his back, causing him to go five days in a row without proper sleep. This led to a flare up of his coronary heart disease and subsequent hospitalization. After his chest oppression, chest pain, and vertigo abated and he was released from the hospital, he decided to seek Chinese medical treatment.

FIRST VISIT: February 3rd, 2009

The patient presents with a sallow, dry complexion and depressed affect. He complains of poor appetite, stomach distention, frequent eructation, a feeling of distention that radiates to the area around DU9 on his back, distention in the lower abdomen, night sweats, and severe insomnia in which he tosses and turns virtually the entire night. His urine and bowel movements are reportedly normal.

71

PULSE: sunken and thin

TONGUE: Thick, white, greasy coating

ABDOMINAL PALPATION: Normal

BACK PALPATION: Pain upon pressing at DU9

After massage, bleeding, and cupping at DU9, the patient began continually eructing with deep, thunderous belches. He reported that after the eructation subsided, he experienced noticeable relief at DU9. I prescribed him five packets of Ba Wei Jie Yu Tang.[6]

SECOND VISIT: February 8th, 2009

The patient reported that his stomach distention, eructation, and distended, blocked feeling at DU9 were all noticeably relieved the day of the last treatment, and he had a very good sleep. The next day, he began taking the herbs and noticed continued improvement of his condition for the next two days. However, on the third day, his symptoms began to relapse, and by the fourth and fifth days, the stomach distention became particularly pronounced around RN17, leading to insomnia. After much consideration, I concluded that his condition resembled liver fixity, a condition described in the *Essential Prescriptions of the Golden Cabinet*, consisting of blood stagnation in the chest and diaphragm. As such, I diagnosed him with a Xuan Fu Hua Tang pattern and prescribed seven packets of Xuan Fu Hua Tang.[7]

THIRD VISIT: March 7th, 2009

---

[6] A formula developed by Huang Huang consisting of Ban Xia Hou Pu Tang plus Si Ni San with Zhi Shi replaced with Zhi Ke.

[7] An Essential Prescriptions of the Golden Cabinet formula composed of Xuan Fu Hua, Cong and Qian Cao. There exists some degree of debate over the mechanism and use of this formula, but it is generally believed to be indicated for cold stagnation of liver blood leading to a feeling of oppression in the chest.

After taking Xuan Fu Hua Tang, all symptoms gradually improved. After taking another twenty packets, the patient reported a near complete resolution of symptoms. Upon follow-up two weeks after suspension of treatment, there had been no relapse of symptoms.

CLINICAL INSIGHT

This was a complicated and deceptive case—the eructation, stomach distention, and counterflow concealed the true cause of disease, which was the liver fixity or blood stagnation in the chest and diaphragm. The patient had a thirty-year history of disease including unresolved dumping syndrome, hypertension, and coronary heart disease, but diagnosis was complicated by the fact that neither his symptomatology nor constitution betrayed any signs of blood stagnation. To a degree, my diagnosis of Xuan Fu Hua Tang was merely a guess. Clearly, we need to continue to research and observe other possible clinical signs and symptoms that would help point to a blood stagnation diagnosis.

Abdominal Pain Treated with Da Jian Zhong Tang

10 YEARS, FEMALE

HISTORY: The patient complained of suffering from severe and frequent abdominal pain for several months. Recently, the pain episodes had become even more frequent, often arising several times in a single day and accompanied by vomiting of stomach acid. A local hospital diagnosed her with ascariasis, but several rounds of antiparasitic medication failed to relieve her symptoms.

CURRENT: The patient's mother reported she is often hypotensive and has cold hands and feet. Additionally, the patient reported having a poor appetite, acid reflux, and alternating sloppy and dry stools.

PULSE: Sunken and weak

TONGUE: Pale with a white coating

ABDOMINAL PALPATION: The abdominal muscles were thick and tight, and upon light palpation, an irregular pattern of bulging protrusions could be felt below the muscle layer, as if there were a small animal slipping around inside her belly. Harder pressure on the abdomen resulted in light pain. Additionally, borborygmus was clearly audible without a stethoscope.

DIAGNOSIS: Tàiyīn disease with replete interior yīn cold. Treatment should focus on warming the middle, supplementing vacuity, descending counterflow, and relieving pain.

FORMULA: Da Jian Zhong Tang: Shu Jiao 4.5g, Gan Jiang 3g, Dang Shen 9g, E Jiao 15g (Three packets)

After taking the herbs, the reflux and abdominal pain completely resolved, and her appetite increased. Upon palpation, I found that the bulging protrusions in her abdomen had vanished.

CLINICAL INSIGHT

The bulging protrusions of the abdomen mentioned in this case are known in modern medicine to be indicative of intestinal obstruction. In children and underweight individuals, these bulges, along with peristaltic waves, are signs of functional pathology. The protrusions are a very important diagnostic sign in intestinal obstruction.

PALPATION METHOD: Have the patient lie supine with their legs unflexed and expose the entire abdomen. Upon observing the superficial appearance of the abdomen, an irregular pattern of protruding bulges of various sizes and lengths can be seen. Some of the protrusions will be a bulge limited to a small area, while others will take on the shape of the intestine. Sometimes the bulges will be limited to a small area, while in other cases they can be seen throughout the stomach. Upon palpation, these bulges are smooth and soft and feel like capsules. Percussion often yields a tympanic sound.

Chronic Colitis Treated with Shen Qi Wan (Kidney yáng deficient type)

MR. HU, 73 YEARS

FIRST VISIT: October 12th, 2000.

The patient reports having suffered from chronic diarrhea for three years. He complains of borborygmus, sloppy stools, and has six to seven bowel movements per day. Every day in the early morning he will have diarrhea. He speaks with a soft voice, and complains of fatigue, cold limbs, weakness, and a lack of desire to talk.

PULSE: Sunken and thin

TONGUE: Dark and pale with a thick white coating.

ABDOMINAL PALPATION: The lower abdomen is soft and lacks springiness, the abdominal muscles of the lower left and lower right quadrants are tense and painful to the touch. Looking over his medical record, I saw that previous doctors had prescribed Si Shen Wan, Fu Zi Li Zhong Tang, and Wei Ling Tang with little success. This was clearly a case of kidney yáng vacuity. The target of treatment is the 'hypertonicity in the lower left and right quadrants" found in the Shen Qi Wan pattern. As such, I prescribed Shen Qi Wan in decoction form.

After taking seven packets, the borborygmus and bowel movement frequency reduced. This confirmed to me that I had diagnosed the pattern correctly, so I continued prescribing Shen Qi Wan, but switched to pills taken twice a day, 10g each. After fifteen days, the patient's energy noticeably recovered, his stools were formed, and he was down to two to three bowel movements per day. I continued prescribing the same formula for one month, slowly chipping away at the illness to arrive at complete resolution. Gradually, his symptoms completely resolved, and he was still in good condition upon follow-up a year later. If he had any slight relapse, he would just take Shen Qi Wan for a few days and his condition would recover.

CLINICAL INSIGHT

There are two different kinds of formulas: "general use" formulas and "disease-targeted" formulas. General use formulas have a wide scope of application but are not specifically tailored to treat any one disease. Conversely, disease-targeted formulas are specifically tailored to treat certain diseases but have a very narrow scope of application. For the elderly, who have deficiencies ranging from yīn and yáng vacuity to qì and blood vacuity, general use formulas might be a better fit than disease targeted formulas. The patient in this case was over seventy years old and had a clear case of kidney yáng vacuity, so based upon the notion that the kidney opens at the two yīn, it would have been logical to conclude that his diarrhea was due to kidney yáng vacuity. Si Shen Wan and Fu Zi Li Zhong Tang are disease-targeted formulas used in kidney yáng vacuity diarrhea. The art of medicine, however, is profound and subtle and no strategy is ever a guaranteed success. If an improper formula is selected, the treatment will be a failure, so we shouldn't limit ourselves to disease-targeted formulas. My success in using Shen Qi Wan in this case helped me realize that when treating the elderly, I ought to consider using more general use formulas.

Chronic Colitis Treated with Fu Zi Li Zhong Tang plus Ling Gui Zhu Gan Tang (Combined Acupuncture and Herbal Treatment)

The patient was a twenty-four-year-old fisherman who had suffered from chronic diarrhea for two years. He had previously been diagnosed with chronic colitis and irritable bowel syndrome, yet a long course of treatment had been unsuccessful. A Chinese medical doctor had treated him based on a diagnosis of large intestine damp-heat but failed to improve his condition. Finally, he resorted to a folk doctor who treated him with toxin-resolving and anti-diarrheal herbs, but this method also proved unhelpful. After trying all these treatment methods and not seeing the slightest bit of improvement, the patient lost any hope of being cured. At that point, a family member of his arranged for me to go treat him at his home. He was apparently unaware of the arrangement and was at first reticent to come downstairs when I arrived. This left me in a bit of an awkward position that was only resolved when his wife forcibly dragged him downstairs to see me. As he reluctantly slumped down the stairs, I immediately noticed his tall, emaciated build, thick cotton sweatpants and sweater, dark, sallow, and malnourished-looking skin, and the look of pure suspicion and wariness written across his face. Yet, despite suffering through years of chronic disease, his eyes still shone brightly with an intelligent glimmer.

I felt deeply sympathetic to his plight—to be so crippled by disease at such a young age must have been very difficult and I just didn't believe that a standard case of colitis couldn't be cured. I listened patiently as he described the course of his disease and treatment over the past two years. I tried to project a sense of understanding and friendliness as he spoke and expressed my sympathy for the difficulties he'd been through.

Gradually, this approach helped to mitigate some of that initial animosity. I noticed that he was very precise and systematic in his description and would adroitly emphasize specific points of interest, but there was also a clear sense of pessimism and despair in his language. After he finished speaking, I had him put his cold, pallid hand on a rolled-up book that I used in place of a pulse-taking pillow.

His pulse was thin, and his tongue was pale red. He complained of feeling cold, cold limbs, vertigo, fatigue, poor appetite, copious saliva, copious clear urine, diarrhea multiple times a day, and mild bowel incontinence. These symptoms were all indicative of tàiyīn and shàoyīn disease and constituted a classic Fu Zi Li Zhong Tang presentation. His abdominal muscles were flat, paper-thin and weak and he had a substernal splash sound and substernal palpitations. These findings were largely consistent with the above diagnosis, but the substernal splashing, palpitations, and vertigo suggested he also had water counterflow. As such, in addition to Fu Zi Li Zhong Tang, he would also need Ling Gui Zhu Gan Tang.

Throughout the diagnosis, the patient maintained a cold, standoffish attitude. This was the first time I had ever encountered such an uncooperative patient. After writing my prescription, I gave him a thorough explanation of my clinical reasoning and instructed him to first take five packets.

I was confident I could cure him, so I smiled and said to him, "As long as you are patient and cooperate with treatment, you will make a full recovery."

"Have you treated something like this before?" He asked.

I could hear in his voice that despite the fact that he didn't completely trust me, he had already let down his guard a bit after hearing my analysis.

I nodded and said with a smile, "I treated a woman in my town who had chronic diarrhea for two years and severe leukorrhea for one year with Fu Zi Li Zhong Tang plus Zhen Wu Tang. I cured her and it only took a little over a month."

He half-believingly replied, "I met many chronic diarrhea patients in the hospital who had very clear diagnoses — allergic colitis, irritable bowel syndrome, intestinal tuberculosis — but none of them got better."

I admitted that what he said was true: "Western medicine is capable of diagnosing various forms of chronic colitis, but their treatment is hit-or-miss. Chinese medicine and acupuncture are much more effective for treating this disease."

He seemed to get emotional and asked, "I've seen many Chinese doctors and taken vats worth of Chinese herbs, so why haven't I gotten better yet?"

I didn't know exactly how to answer that question, so I said: "Chinese medicine doesn't have a specific formula for treating chronic colitis, treatment will only be effective with accurate diagnosis and formula pattern identification."

"How do you know that your diagnosis is correct?" He asked, without the slightest pretense of politeness.

"The formula pattern method used in The *Treatise on Cold Damage* is the most effective method of treatment that Chinese medicine has to offer." I realized that I'd have to spell it all out for him, so I continued, saying, "Your symptom presentation conforms to the shàoyīn disease Fu Zi Li Zhong Tang pattern and the tàiyīn disease Ling Gui Zhu Gan Tang pattern." I then went on to compare his symptom presentation with the principal symptoms in shàoyīn and tàiyīn disease and showed how his symptomology and abdominal presentation corresponded to the Fu Zi Li Zhong Tang and Ling Gui Zhu Gan Tang patterns. He didn't say a word throughout my explanation and his eyes seemed to shine with ardent interest.

"Ultimately, the only way to establish whether diagnosis was accurate is by taking the herbs. If you're willing to try, you can start by taking five packets." I said.

I then handed him the following prescription: Zhi Gan Cao 6g, Fu Zi 9g, Bai Zhu 15g, Dang Shen 15g, Gui Zhi 9g, Fu Ling 15g, Gan Jiang 9g. (Five packets)

He studied the prescription for quite some time and didn't say a word. I could see that he was still a bit hesitant, so I told him that before taking the medicine, we could start by having him do moxibustion for one week. I instructed him to moxa at RN12, RN6, RN4, and SP9 and explained to him that performing moxa at these points would warm and supplement tàiyīn and shàoyīn yángqì, and warm, unblock and disperse pathological water throughout the body in a similar fashion to Fu Zi Li Zhong Tang and Ling Gui Zhu Gan Tang. Even if the diagnosis were incorrect, there wouldn't be any serious side effects, but if the moxa was helpful, I suggested we could use a combination of moxa and herbs to speed up his recovery.

This combination of clear and practical analysis of the formula pattern together with my offer to let him first moxa and then take herbs and my warm and confident demeanor finally overcame the patient's cynicism and reluctance and he gladly assented to my treatment plan. Through that long and rather difficult process, I finally got my first patient in the town of Zhuang Yuan.

One week later, he arrived at my clinic with a big smile on his face. After just one week of moxibustion, he felt a sense of ease and comfort in his body that he hadn't felt for years, his symptoms had all improved and his bowel incontinence was greatly reduced. The positive results had reinforced his trust in me, and he obligingly took home a week of herbs to continue treatment. After taking the herbs, he continued to improve, so I stayed with the same formula and recommended that he continue using moxibustion every day. After three continuous months of treatment, all symptoms resolved with the exception of some fatigue and weakness.

CLINICAL INSIGHT

Performing moxa at RN12, RN6, RN4, and SP9 warms and supplements tàiyīn and shàoyīn yángqì, and warms, unblocks and disperses pathological water throughout the body in a manner similar to Fu Zi Li Zhong

Tang plus Ling Gui Zhu Gan Tang. Using moxa and herbs in tandem yields "twice the effect for half the effort".

Gastroenteritis Treated with Ban Xia Xie Xin Tang

The first patient I ever prescribed a formula for was a young farmer in our commune's work unit. After eating too many eggs and rice dumplings during the dragon boat festival celebrations, he began suffering from stomach pain, diarrhea, and vomiting. He was diagnosed with gastroenteritis by a local hospital and did recover to a degree after treatment, however he continued to experience stomach distension, sloppy stools, and vomiting that failed to resolve after several months. The Chinese doctors he saw diagnosed him with food damage, but the formulas they gave, which all revolved around abductive dispersion and transforming food, were not only ineffective, but they also actually exacerbated his condition. In just three months, he lost 20kg. Having exhausted his options, he came to me looking for help. Based upon his three main symptoms — substernal hard glomus, vomiting and nausea, and borborygmus with diarrhea, I concluded he had a Ban Xia Xie Xin Tang formula pattern.

"When there is vomiting, borborygmus, and substernal glomus, Ban Xia Xie Xin Tang is indicated." This is the classic description of the symptom and sign presentation for Ban Xia Xie Xin Tang found in the *Essential Prescriptions of the Golden Cabinet*. This illustrates that the formula pattern presents in the upper, middle and lower thirds of the body: vomiting above, glomus in the middle, and borborygmus below — manifesting symptoms throughout the entire GI tract. Given that the patient also had canker sores and insomnia, I ended up going with Gan Cao Xie Xin Tang. At the time, I was young and confident, and I was sure that the formula would be effective because the patient's symptoms perfectly matched the formula pattern. After taking three packets, his symptoms noticeably improved and I was overjoyed. I knew I had found a system that worked and was worthy of further study. After around a month of treatment, the farmer's condition completely resolved.

In treating this patient's food damage, I didn't use a single abductive dispersion or food transforming herb and, yet, I was still able to completely resolve his gastroenteritis. To this day, forty years later, I still keep in touch with that patient. I will always remember that case because the success I had cemented my belief in the power of Zhang Zhong-jing's *Treatise on Cold Damage* and showed me how formula pattern identification could guide my clinical process.

I should emphasize that I'm not categorically opposed to using abductive dispersion or food transforming herbs in food damage patients. Quite the opposite, whenever I encounter patients that have a Bao He Wan formula pattern, an abductive dispersion formula, I prescribe Bao He Wan without the slightest hesitation. The formula pattern for Bao He Wan is halitosis, aversion to food, eructation and reflux, elicitation of pain and avoidance upon pressing the abdomen, incomplete bowel movements with malodorous stools, and a sticky, greasy tongue coating.

Pediatric Chronic Cough Treated with Bao He Wan

A six-year-old girl who was the daughter of the director of the resident's committee in the neighborhood I used to live in suffered from a chronic cough that had failed to respond to over a year of treatment. When she came to me for treatment, I noticed her symptoms and signs were completely in line with the Bao He Wan formula pattern: halitosis, malodorous stools, yellow urine, aversion to food, abdominal distention and discomfort, a greasy yellow tongue coating, etc. Given the correspondence, I prescribed her three packets of Bao He Wan. Two days later, the resident committee director called me up all upset and said:

"She's taken the medicine for two days now. The first day was fine, but today she's already had diarrhea three times. What is going on?"

"Are her bowel movements particularly stinky?" I asked.

"They're nearly unbearable." He replied.

"How is her cough?" I asked.

Then it suddenly dawned on him: "I haven't heard her cough at all today!"

"Then there's no problem. Make sure she takes the last packet." I said.

With that, the little girl's chronic cough, which hadn't responded to over a year of treatment, was cured.

Coldness of the Toes Accompanied by Abdominal Discomfort and Diarrhea Treated with Gui Zhi Jia Fu Zi Tang

50 YEARS, MALE (FARMER)

HISTORY: The patient had previously always been in good health and claims to have never had any serious illness in the past. However, for the past five years, he would often feel coldness in his toes, especially in the summer. As soon as his toes would go cold, he would begin to feel abdominal discomfort followed shortly by diarrhea. This year, these episodes have become more frequent, and he's also started to develop spasms in his arms and legs. He had never had spasms like this before and they were causing him great concern. He had been to the hospital several times and seen many different doctors, but they all concluded that he had irritable bowel syndrome, and their treatments were ineffective. The patient is a distant relative of mine and upon hearing that I was a doctor through our family, he came to see me at my clinic.

FIRST VISIT: July 10th, 2005

Apart from the above symptoms, the patient also complained of night sweats in the winter, spontaneous sweating in the summer, copious saliva, and lack of thirst. His pulse and tongue, however, seemed normal. Upon abdominal palpation, I found his abdominal muscles to be thin and weak. I originally considered using Gui Zhi Tang, but then I remembered an experience rhyme by a *kampo* practitioner that recommended Gui Zhi Jia Fu Zi Tang for abdominal pain in the summer with cold feet. As such, I decided to prescribe seven packets of Gui Zhi Jia Fu Zi Tang substituting Sheng Jiang for Gan Jiang, thereby making the formula a combination of Gui Zhi Tang and Si Ni Tang.

After one week of herbs, the patient returned on July 17th. He reported that nearly as soon as he took the medicine, he felt a full-body sense of ease and comfort, along with a joyous feeling as if he had suddenly run into an old friend he hadn't seen for a long time. The coldness in his feet accompanied by episodes of diarrhea also diminished. Because the previous formula seemed to have worked well, I gave him another seven packets.

After another week of herbs, the curative effects of the formula began to manifest: the spasms had completely resolved and the cold feet with diarrhea episodes had noticeably reduced. However, the patient still complained of spontaneous sweating. Based upon the above symptoms, I prescribed the original formula plus Yu Ping Feng San and asked him to take it for another two weeks and then stop and monitor symptoms.

The patient continued to take the formula for another month, after which all symptoms subsided. When I met up with some of his family members a year later, they informed me that he hadn't had any relapse of symptoms.

CLINICAL INSIGHT

Experience rhymes in the jīngfāng tradition should be taken seriously. In Zen Buddhism, there is a notion of transmission of knowledge outside of formal writing[8]—the same concept applies in the realm of medicine. In the "Comprehending the Root" chapter of the *Baopuzi* (抱朴子) it states, "Many of the most important concepts (in cultivation) are not

---

[8] 直指人心，見性成佛，教外別傳，不立文字。 From the Bodhidharma's *Sermon on Awakening*. This quote originally derives from a purported historical event in which Sakyamuni buddha gave a wordless sermon to his disciples by holding up a white flower. Mahaskyapa was the only disciple to understand the meaning of his sermon. The buddha then said: "I possess the true *Dharma* eye, the marvelous mind of Nirvana, the true form of the formless, the subtle *dharma* gate that does not rest on words or letters but is a special transmission outside of the scriptures. This I entrust to Mahākāśyapa." Dr. Lou is using this quote as a means of saying that the poems and rhymes are a "special transmission outside of the scriptures".

written in the daoist scriptures and writings on immortality. The only way to learn such sacred knowledge is to make sacrificial offerings at altars, then the poems will be taught to you." The Tang dynasty poet Cen Shen once recalled, "As a boy, I was fond of internal alchemy and was once taught experience rhymes from a Daoist practitioner." The distinguishing characteristic of jīngfāng medicine is its emphasis on treating based on pattern, identifying formulas that correspond to pattern presentations, and distinguishing between patterns. In the above case, it would have been difficult to discern a clear disease etiology and mechanism. However, by employing formula pattern diagnosis combined with a *kampo* experience rhyme, I easily arrived at an effective treatment strategy. Why wouldn't other clinical physicians adopt this strategy?

Why didn't I consider adding Xi Xin to treat this patient's cold feet? Xi Xin treats deeply lodged rheum and congested fluid, which is why it is used to treat substernal pathologic water with cough and fullness. This patient felt cold, had cold limbs, excessive sweating, and diarrhea. This is a classic Si Ni Tang pattern, which is why I added Fu Zi and switched out Sheng Jiang for Gan Jiang to ensure the formula corresponded to the pattern.

Night Sweats, Nocturnal Emissions and Excessive Dreaming Treated with Gui Zhi Jia Long Gu Mu Li Tang

30 YEARS, MALE

HISTORY: The patient has suffered from night sweats, nocturnal emissions, and excessive dreaming for several years and has responded poorly to a wide variety of treatments. In recent months, his condition has worsened, so he came seeking treatment at my clinic.

FIRST VISIT: January 24th, 2003

The patient is tall, relatively thin, has a pallid complexion, and looks rather fatigued. Apart from the above symptoms, he also complains of a heavy feeling in his head, headache, a feeling of heat radiating from his head, aversion to wind and cold, constipation, and yellow urine, etc.

ABDOMINAL PALPATION: Substernal glomus and fullness and a 2–3cm long induration in the periphery of his lower abdomen next to the navel that felt like mechanical pencil lead.

The above symptoms in combination with this abdominal presentation constitute a classic Gui Zhi Jia Long Gu Mu Li Tang pattern. As such, I first prescribed ten packets of Gui Zhi Jia Long Gu Mu Li Tang. After four or five days taking the herbs, the patient reported that the aversion to wind and cold and the head symptoms gradually receded. After five to six days, the night sweats and dreaming reduced and he'd had only one nocturnal emission. Upon abdominal palpation, I noted that his substernal glomus and fullness and periumbilical induration were reduced. However, the patient still complained of fatigue and heaviness in the limbs which was relieved by lying down.

Based on these symptoms, I added 10g of Dang Shen and 20g of Bai Shao and prescribed a month's worth of herbs. He never came back to the clinic, but I ran into him on the street 6 months later and he told me that he was completely back to normal. When I asked him about the pencil lead induration in his stomach, he said it was still there, but much less pronounced than before.

Clinical Insight

Abdominal palpation diagnosis is extremely important. Tōdō Yoshimasu believed that the abdominal presentation was more important than any other symptoms or signs. Despite being a local symptomatic manifestation, the abdominal presentation can reflect the state of the entire organism. As such, formulas and acumoxa treatment styles that are correlated with abdominal presentations can exert their regulatory effect on the body as whole. In Korean medicine, there is also a special approach to treatment called "treating (via) the abdomen".

Gui Zhi Jia Long Gu Mu Li Tang's main abdominal presentation, "Tight rigidity in the lower left and right quadrants", can manifest in two ways in clinic: 1.) An induration that feels like pencil lead can be felt upon palpation next to or below the umbilicus right below the skin layer. In *Compendium of Key Techniques in Massage* (厘正按摩要術), the Qing Dynasty physician Zhang Zhen-jian (張振鑒) clearly stated: "Above and below the umbilicus is the realm of the Ren channel. If a chopstick-like induration is palpated in this area, it is a sign of spleen and kidney vacuity." In *Thirty Years of Kampo Medicine Practice* (漢方診療三十年), Keisetsu Ōtsuka (大冢敬節) stated, "Beside the umbilicus, a 2–3cm induration resembling pencil lead can be found in a Gui Zhi Jia Long Gu Mu Li Tang pattern." 2.) In his *Introduction to Clinical Formulas* (中醫臨證處方入門), Kazuo Tatsuno (龍野一雄) commented: "Tight rigidity refers to the tightness of the rectus abdominus in the lower abdomen, but "tight rigidity" implies severe tightness. This level of tightness can be found in the Gui Zhi Jia Long Gu Mu Li Tang pattern."

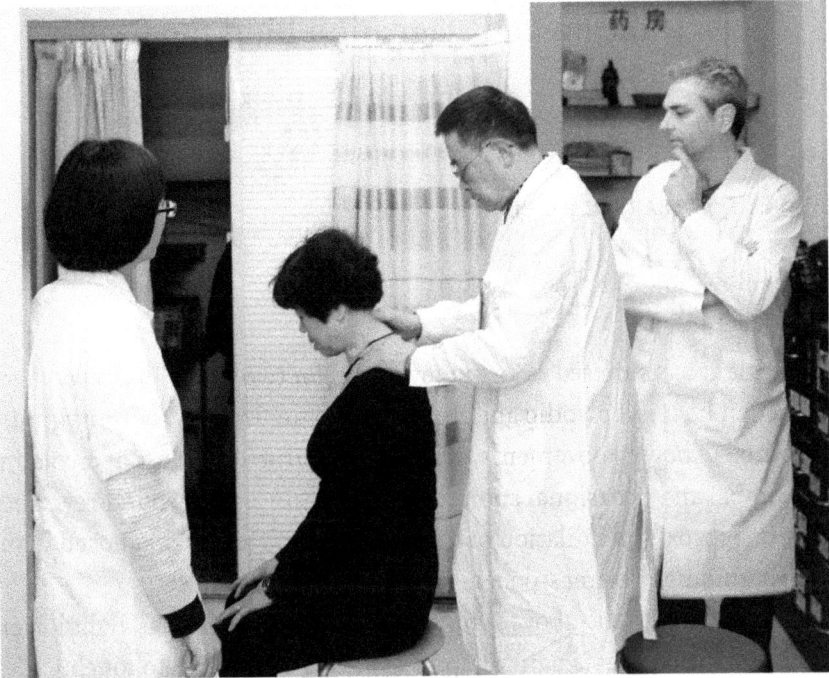

PICTURED: Dr. Lou in his home clinic with his two students

Ureter Stone Treated with Da Huang Fu Zi Tang plus Shao Yao Gan Cao Tang (Phlegm and stagnation bind type)

MR. WU, 50 YEARS (CADRE)

FIRST VISIT: July 28th, 1998

The patient has suffered from kidney stones for two years. Three days ago, he began having episodic abdominal pain and urgency, borborygmus, incomplete bowel movements, scant, yellow urine, coldness and cold in the limbs, and occasional spontaneous sweating. Ultrasound revealed hydronephrosis and dilation of the right ureter. He was diagnosed with a right middle ureteral stone.

In addition to the above symptoms, the patient also has right lower back distention that is painful upon knocking and averse to touch.

PULSE: Wiry, tight, and forceful

TONGUE: Dark and pale with a white, greasy coating and phlegm-like substance above the coating

ABDOMINAL PALPATION: The entire abdomen is distended, full, and upon pressing feels tight and constricted. The area from below the right rib line to the side of the navel is glomular, hard, and painful upon firm pressing.

DIAGNOSIS: This is phlegm and stagnation congealing into stones. The presentation closely conforms to a tàiyīn Da Huang Fu Zi Tang plus Shao Yao Gan Cao Tang pattern:

Sheng Da Huang 10g (put in towards end of decoction), Fu Zi 10g (decoct before other herbs), Xi Xin 3g, Bai Shao 30g, Zhi Gan Cao 6g. (Two packets) (Boil herbs on high heat and drink decoction down quickly)

After taking the herbs, the patient's abdominal distention and fullness gradually subsided and he was able to pass urine and bowel movements normally. He felt a full-body sense of comfort and desired sleep. Three days later, he took another dose, after which all symptoms completely resolved. His lower back no longer exhibited knocking pain and his abdomen returned to normal. Upon follow-up two years later, he reported there had been no relapse of symptoms.

CLINICAL INSIGHT

This case of ureter stone was due to phlegm and stagnation bind that congealed into stones in the context of prolonged cold. The patient's abdominal pain, coldness of limbs, pale dark tongue, greasy tongue coating, and tight and wiry pulse are all clear signs of cold. The abdominal aversion to touch, lower-back knocking pain, blocked urine and bowel movements, and forceful pulse are all signs of a replete condition. The rib-side pain, rigidity of the abdominal muscles, episodic spasmodic pain, and tight pulse were all clear signs of a Da Huang Fu Zi Tang[9] plus Shao Yao Gan Cao Tang pattern.

---

[9] Pain below the rib on one side that radiates downward is a classic Da Huang Fu Zi Tang abdominal pattern.

Postoperative Urinary Retention Treated with Shen Qi Wan (Kidney Yáng Type)

After cervical spine surgery, the patient developed post-operative urinary retention. Having spent over 17 days as an in-patient, he was first intermittently catheterized, but later developed a urinary tract infection, after which there was no choice but to put him on a long-term catheter. The hospital eventually decided to transfer him to a larger hospital in Shanghai. When he arrived in Shanghai, he requested to see a Chinese doctor.

CURRENT: The patient appears to be in low spirits, is fatigued, and has a sallow complexion. He complains of full-body joint pain, numbness in the limbs, aversion to cold, and excessive dreaming. Urine and bowel movements are normal.

PULSE: Sunken and thin

TONGUE: Engorged and pale red with a thick, white, moist coating.

ABDOMINAL PALPATION: Tight rigidity in the lower left and right abdominal quadrants, below the navel palpation yields a bind about the width of pencil lead.

DIAGNOSIS: This is a case of kidney yáng vacuity with dysfunctional urinary bladder qì transformation.

TREATMENT: needle RN4 and RN3, Shen Qi Wan in decoction form (two packets).

I advised the patient to remove their catheter in advance and use Deng Xin Cao to prick the inside of the nose to induce sneezing, which would increase intra-abdominal pressure and promote the passing of urine. The patient was initially hesitant, but eventually decided to remove the catheter. Five hours after taking the medicine, he felt urinary urgency and used the above method to induce sneezing, after which he was able to pass urine himself.

On his second visit, I advised him to take 10g of Shen Qi Wan in pill form twice daily for two weeks. He reported that after taking that regime, the urinary retention completely resolved. Upon follow-up one year later, he said he hadn't had any relapses.

CLINICAL INSIGHT

Despite this being an acute and severe illness, treatment still only required the "turning" or transformation of kidney qì. As the *Golden Mirror of Medicine* (醫宗金鑑) remarks regarding qì aspect pathology in the *Essential Prescriptions of the Golden Cabinet*: "When defense and construction qi are blocked, (water) qì accumulates in the bladder. The defense and construction qì are both taxed, resulting in encumbered qi on the exterior and a cold body, while in the interior, blocked qì leads to pain in the bones. When qì is able to communicate between the interior and exterior, qì flow is restored. With this "turning" of the great qì, (water) qì is dispersed." From this statement it is quite clear that the notion in Chinese medicine that "the kidney and urinary bladder govern qi transformation" is not some whimsical statement. The focus of diagnosis in this treatment was on the abdominal presentation: as soon as I palpated the pencil-lead line directly below the navel I knew this was a Shen Qi Wan pattern.

Shen Qi Wan is primarily a kidney yáng supplementing formula but also includes elements of yīn-yáng dual supplementation. In Japan, this formula is known as the primary formula for treating diseases of the elderly. In China, some people are hesitant to use the formula because it contains Fu Zi and Rou Gui, but this is overblown. Together, Rou Gui and Fu Zi constitute only 1/8 of the dose of Di Huang, a formula structure that embodies the *Inner Classic* idea of "gentle fire engenders qì." As long as one diagnoses this formula pattern correctly, it is sure to be effective. In this regard, abdominal palpation is extremely important. Despite being a local symptomatic manifestation, the abdominal presentation can reflect the state of the entire organism. As such, formulas and acumoxa treatment styles that are correlated with abdominal presentations can exert their regulatory effect on the body as a whole.

Zhong-jing described the Shen Qi Wan abdominal presentation in terms of "insensitivity of the left and right lower abdominal quadrants" and "tightness and rigidity of the lower left and right quadrants". In actual clinical practice, this pattern can manifest in three ways: 1.) Numbness in the lower left and right quadrants, 2.) Rigidity of the rectus abdominus in lower left and right quadrants, 3.) A pencil lead-like knot below the navel. In *Compendium of Key Techniques in Massage*, the Qing Dynasty physician Zhang Zhen-jian clearly stated: "Above and below the umbilicus is the realm of the Ren channel. If a chopstick-like induration is palpated in this area, it is a sign of spleen and kidney vacuity." In *The Classic of Clinical Kampo Diagnosis and Treatment* (臨床應用漢方診療醫典) Keisetsu Ōtsuka calls this presentation the "middle line pith" and gives a detailed description: "some middle line piths run from above the navel all the way through it and down below the navel. Some are restricted to just above or below the navel. If the pith is only palpable below the navel, this is an indicator for using Ba Wei Wan." This is a clear and incisive portrayal of clinical reality. In cases of kidney yáng vacuity with this classic abdominal presentation, Shen Qi Wan should be the first choice.

Lower Back Pain and Aversion to Cold Treated with Xiao Xian Xiong Tang plus Ge Gen Tang plus Shao Yao (Herniated Disk)

MR. J, 56 YEARS (170CM, 70KG)

FIRST VISIT: October 15th, 2014

CC: Lower back pain and aversion to cold for years

HISTORY: Lower back pain that is worsened by cold weather. The patient has tried many forms of treatment with no success. Last year, a regimen of Shen Zhuo Tang temporarily reduced the pain, but caused a splitting headache and insomnia. The previous doctor thought he must have non-interaction of the heart and kidney and gave him Jiao Tai Wan plus Fu Zi Xie Xin Tang with underwhelming results. He was diagnosed with 4th and 5th lumbar HIVD.

CURRENT: The patient has an average build and claims to have a balanced diet. Apart from his back pain, he does not admit having any other symptoms.

ABDOMINAL PALPATION: Rectus abdominus is tight and contracted with moderate springiness, and there is substernal pain upon pressing. He complains of rigidity in his neck and the lower back is cool and damp to the touch.

DIAGNOSIS: This is a Xiao Xiang Xiong Tang plus Ge Gen Tang plus Shao Yao formula pattern.

FORMULA: Ge Gen 60g, Ma Huang 5g, Gui Zhi 20g, Bai Shao 15g, Chi Shao 15g, Sheng Jiang 5 slices, Gan Cao 5g, Hong Zao 5 pieces, Ban Xia 10g, Huang Lian 5g, Gua Lou Ren 10g, Gua Lou Pi 10g. (Seven packets, one per day)

SECOND VISIT: October 23rd

The patient reported that after taking two packets of herbs, his condition worsened, and he was in bed for a week before pain slowly began to subside. His abdominal presentation showed signs of progress.

FORMULA: Ge Gen 60g, Ma Huang 5g, Gui Zhi 20g, Bai Shao 15g, Chi Shao 15g, Sheng Jiang 5 slices, Gan Cao 5g, Da Zao 5 pieces, Ban Xia 10g, Huang Lian 5g, Gua Lou Ren 10g, Gua Lou Pi 10g. (Twelve packets, one per day. Rest one day after taking six packets)

Upon follow-up six months later, he said the HIVD had completely resolved and hadn't relapsed since.

Ge Gen Tang is effective in treating nerve pain, rheumatoid arthritis, and HIVD of the cervical and lumbar spine—I have a large number of cases in which I've used Ge Gen Tang to treat these diseases with success. Of course, in clinic we should never limit ourselves to just using one formula to treat a certain disease. We must go into every case with an open and clear mind and prescribe based upon formula pattern correspondence.

When using Ge Gen Tang to treat pain due to muscular spasm or convulsion, a heavy dose of Ge Gen must be used, anywhere from 30 to 60g on average. Oftentimes, a heavier dose of Bai Shao or Bai Shao and Chi Shao combined is needed. In most of these cases, I dose Gui Zhi at 15–20g, too little will yield poor results. When taking Ge Gen Tang, mìnxuàn reactions like exacerbation of joint and back pain are common, so you must inform patients ahead of time to avoid patients thinking you prescribed the wrong formula.

Abdominal diagnosis is the key to prescription. If I hadn't used abdominal palpation, I never would have arrived at a diagnosis of a Xiao Xian Xiong Tang pattern. If I hadn't combined the Ge Gen Tang with Xiao Xian Xiong Tang, the patient might have developed a headache and insomnia like he did with the previous formula. This would cause the patient to abandon treatment before the herbs had time to act.

Bell's Palsy Treated with Ge Gen Tang

Ms. Wang, 75 years

The patient reports that around three months ago, she felt numbness in the right side of her face upon waking up one morning and would drip water from the right side of her mouth when rinsing her mouth. Additionally, she complained of a loss of taste, inability to close her right eye, and numbness in the right side of her tongue. When eating, her tongue movement was impaired, and food would gather in her right cheek. She had a dark, sallow complexion and complained of near constant aversion to cold, heat effusion, and lack of sweating. She also complained of bitterness in the mouth, stomach discomfort for one month, constipation (one BM every three days), distention and pain below the mastoid process at SJ17, and pain upon pressing at DU9.

TONGUE: Red with a yellow coating

PULSE: Floating and tight

ABDOMINAL PALPATION: Substernal pain upon pressing, fullness and discomfort in the chest and rib-side, and full, strong abdominal muscles.

DIAGNOSIS: Tàiyáng shàoyáng dragover disease, Ge Gen Tang and Da Chai Hu Tang formula pattern.

The *kampo* master Ken Fujihara (藤平健) notes that in tàiyáng shàoyáng dragover disease, one can first treat tàiyáng, so I started her with three packets of Ge Gen Tang.

Two months later, the patient brought a friend to my clinic for treatment. I noticed that her palsy was completely healed, so I asked her how she had done with the medicine.

She said, "After taking the first packet, the next day the palsy was completely resolved, so I didn't take the second and third packets."

I asked her, "Why didn't you keep taking the medicine to reinforce the treatment?"

Her reply caught me off guard: "At first my mouth was skewed to the left, but then after just one packet it was corrected. If I took another packet, wouldn't it skew to the right?"

I didn't know if I should laugh or cry.

The reason I didn't combine Ge Gen Tang with Da Chai Hu Tang in this case requires a careful investigation of three yīn three yáng theory in the *Treatise on Cold Damage* as well as an understanding of the rules for treating combination disease and dragover disease. This involves investigating primary symptoms, secondary symptoms, urgent versus chronic symptoms, and root versus branch symptoms.

Trigeminal Neuralgia Treated with Ma Huang Tang

The patient was a middle-aged woman, one of my student's aunts, who had suffered from trigeminal neuralgia for seven years. During episodes, she would experience severe pain in her upper and lower teeth as well as at her temples. During the day, the pain was relatively dull, but at night it would become pronounced and lead to insomnia. During the intake, she complained of aversion to wind, feeling agitated and hot, and rarely sweating. Her pulse was floating and tight. Based on these symptoms, I concluded she had an exterior pattern and prescribed her one packet of Ma Huang Tang.

Early the next morning, shortly after I woke up, I heard a banging on the door and upon opening it, I saw the woman with the trigeminal neuralgia standing there on my stoop. To my shock, she said she hadn't slept a wink the entire previous night.

"How is the pain in your teeth?" I asked.

"Strangely, I haven't had any pain in my teeth and temples today." She replied.

"When did you take the medicine?" I asked her.

"I took the first dose at 8pm and the second dose at 11pm." She said.

"You waited the right amount of time in between doses, but you started taking it too late. You probably were experiencing a side effect from the stimulatory effect of Ma Huang."

Based upon her symptoms, I prescribed her 3 doses of Si Ni San and let blood at EX-HN5. I told her that if she had any relapse of symptoms, she could come back to my clinic any time. She lived on an island off the coast of Wenzhou, so I never heard from her after that. One year later, when I asked my student how she was doing, he said she never had a relapse of symptoms.

This case helped me realize that miscellaneous diseases often include an element of external contraction. If there is an element of exterior contraction, and it isn't addressed, it might be hard to resolve the condition because external contraction is a whole-body pathology, and its influence can be much more powerful than local pathologies.

Trigeminal Neuralgia Treated with Gui Zhi Jia Fu Zi Tang

The patient was a 78-year-old man who arrived at my clinic escorted by his two daughters. He reported that he had previously suffered from trigeminal neuralgia for three years, but after surgery at a local hospital, his condition had been stable for five years. However, the trigeminal nerve pain resurfaced 6 months ago, and he had to take the anti-convulsant drug carbamazepine twice a day just to function. Despite taking the pain killers, there would still be a three-hour period during the night when the pain would become very intense. However, if he tried to take another dose of the carbamazepine during that time, he would become extremely dizzy, so he didn't dare take that third dose. For the past six months, he had tried many different treatments, but none of them had yielded any results. With no other options available, he decided to give Chinese medicine a try.

FIRST VISIT: May 25th, 2009

The patient has a tall, gaunt build and pallid complexion. He complains of aversion to cold, coldness of the limbs, excessive sweating from his head and neck, and he seemed to be quite anxious. He had previously suffered from stomach pain, but ever since developing trigeminal neuralgia, the pain had subsided.

PULSE: Moderate and large

TONGUE: Engorged, scalloped and pale red with a thin white coating.

ABDOMINAL PALPATION: Thin and tight abdominal muscles with a contracted rectus abdominus.

This is a classic Gui Zhi Jia Fu Zi Tang abdominal presentation. So, I prescribed him one week of Gui Zhi Jia Fu Zi Tang. I also needled at EX-HN5 and TH17 with strong stimulation. The needling alone was quite effective in alleviating his pain. I also advised him to continue taking the anticonvulsant at the same dose.

Gui Zhi 10g, Bai Shao 10g, Gan Cao 6g, Da Huang 30g, Sheng Jiang 3 slices, Fu Zi 10g.

SECOND VISIT: June 2nd

The patient reported that the nighttime pain had reduced to two hours and the severity of the pain had also reduced noticeably. He was very happy and felt quite confident that treatment would be successful.

Based upon his feedback, I prescribed another week of Gui Zhi Jia Fu Zi Tang and performed the same acupuncture protocol as the first visit. Over the ensuing course of treatment, his pain gradually subsided, his sleep and appetite improved, and he felt much more energetic. During this process, he also gradually reduced the dose of carbamazepine and weaned off it completely after two months. He eventually stopped needing the acupuncture treatment and switched to taking herbs every other day. One month later, I told him he could stop taking herbs entirely and contact me if there was any relapse.

In the ensuing two years, he had one relapse that presented as a Chai Hu pattern which I resolved using a Xiao Chai Hu Tang modification. After that, he never had another relapse again. Years later, I ran into him while walking to the food market and he informed me that his inguinal hernia had also resolved during the course of treatment.

CLINICAL INSIGHT

Trigeminal neuralgia is a form of headache, so any method used to treat headache can also be used to treat trigeminal neuralgia.

The primary formulas for headache in the *Treatise on Cold Damage* are Ma Huang Tang and Gui Zhi Tang. Despite this being abundantly clear from the text itself, I originally didn't understand this in my early days as a physician. Lines 13 and 35 both start with, "In tàiyáng disease with headache" and both show how Ma Huang Tang and Gui Zhi Tang can be applied to effectively treat both headache and trigeminal neuralgia.

Of the many formula patterns implicated in treating trigeminal neuralgia, Wu Ling San and Wu Zhu Yu Tang also bear mentioning, but I won't go into the details of those patterns here. Certain post-classical formulas like Xuan Qi Tang, Gou Teng San, Qing Shang Chu Tong Tang, and Ban Xia Bai Zhu Tian Ma Tang of course also have their applications. As long as the formula pattern corresponds to the symptom presentation, it will surely be effective. Xuan Qi Tang, a formula from Li Dong-yuan's *Secret Treasure of the Orchid Chamber* (蘭室秘藏) consisting of Huang Qin 6g, Qiang Huo 12g, Fang Feng 12g, Gan Cao 6g, and Ban Xia 15g, primarily treats ophthalmic branch trigeminal nerve pain. The ophthalmic branch innervates the eyebrow among other places, which is precisely the area that Xuan Qi Tang targets. As a result, this formula can often produce marvelous results in the treatment of trigeminal neuralgia.

Full-Body Joint Pain Treated with Gui Zhi Jia Fu Zi Tang

The patient is a 50-year-old female farmer with an average build and a slightly sallow complexion. She reports having suffered from full-body joint pain for one year, which is particularly pronounced in her elbow and knee joints. She lives in a remote mountain community with non-existent medical facilities, so her condition has never been properly treated. In recent months, her condition has worsened, so she came to my clinic for treatment based on a recommendation.

She reports that she has pain in her elbow and knee joints that is worse with cold. There is no redness or swelling observable in the joints. At night, when lying down, the pain is less intense, but she reports having night sweats. She has a slight fever of 38°C, but no cough or rhinorrhea. Her urine, bowel movements, and sleep are all normal.

PULSE: Floating and rapid

TONGUE: pale with a thick white coating.

Based upon the above symptoms and signs, I prescribed Gui Zhi j Fu Zi Tang.

SECOND VISIT: November 18th, 2011

The patient's fever subsided, but the pain in the joints not only failed to improve, it actually worsened. I had warned her that the pain might intensify at first, so she was well-prepared and still willing to come down from the mountain to continue treatment.

Based upon the above symptoms and signs, I prescribed seven packets of the *Essential Prescriptions of the Golden Cabinet* formula Bai Zhu Fu Zi Tang and treated her using acupuncture and wet cupping. After finishing the second prescription and receiving acupuncture, her full-body joint pain improved, and she felt less aversion to cold in her knee and elbow joints. She was very happy with the results and felt even more confident and hopeful that she could make a complete recovery.

I quickly followed up with another prescription of Bai Zhu Fu Zi Tang, adding Huang Qi 30g and Dang Gui 30g. Additionally, I continued using acupuncture and wet cupping. Because it was difficult for the patient to make frequent trips from her home in the mountains, I told her she could stay at home and apply moxa to her knees and elbows every day for one hour. I also asked her to continue taking Bai Zhu Fu Zi Tang plus Huang Qi and Dang Gui for one month.

On a follow-up one year later, the patient reported that after taking the formula for three months and using moxa every day, the pain in her knees and elbows completely subsided. However, the pain came back again recently after coming down with a cold. I first treated her with Gui Zhi Jia Fu Zi Tang and then followed up with Bai Zhu Fu Zi Tang plus Huang Qi 30g, Dang Gui 30g. After one month, her symptoms resolved and haven't relapsed since.

CLINICAL INSIGHT

Modern Chinese medicine often uses wind, cold, and damp-dispelling Qiang Huo and Du Huo as the primary herbs for treating joint pain. By contrast, jīngfāng medicine uses a formula pattern identification treatment strategy centered around Gui Zhi, Bai Zhu, and Fu Zi formula patterns. This disparity in usage reflects the unique characteristics of these two different streams of Chinese medicine.

The *Essential Prescriptions of the Golden Cabinet* formula Bai Zhu Fu Zi Tang is the same as the *Treatise on Cold Damage* formula Gui Zhi Fu Zi qu Gui Jia Bai Zhu Tang. What does this tell us that the same formula went by different names in these two books? Certain *kampo* practitioners believe this shows that the *Golden Cabinet* and the *Treatise* were written by different authors. Another example is the *Golden Cabinet* formula Gua Lou Gui Zhi Tang, which should be written as Gui Zhi Jia Gua Lou Tang based upon the *Treatise*'s naming conventions.

Epilepsy Treated with Modified
Zhen Wu Tang plus Wu Ling San
(Phlegm clouding the heart orifice type)

MR. WANG, 33 YEARS (CADRE)

FIRST VISIT: March 15th, 1995

HISTORY: The patient suffered from frequent unprovoked fainting and convulsions for five years. He was diagnosed with epilepsy via neurological diagnostic testing.

CURRENT: The patient is quite thin and has a pallid complexion. He complains of occasional abdominal pain, sloppy stools with sticky exudate, edema of the lower limbs, and inhibited, scant, yellow urine. During seizures, he first will feel his back suddenly go cold, then he will lose consciousness and go into convulsions with his jaw clenched tight and expectoration of white foam. His seizures typically last 5–10 minutes and he reports feeling cold and dizzy afterwards with palpitations and occasional shivering.

TONGUE: Pale, dark, engorged and tender with a thin, white, greasy coating.

PULSE: Sunken and wiry.

ABDOMEN: Paper-thin abdominal muscles, flat stomach, rigidity in the rectus abdominus, substernal palpitation, and noticeable pulsation upon palpation above the navel.

DIAGNOSIS: This is a case of tàiyīn-shàoyīn combination disease, yáng qì vacuity, and counterflow of rheum-water clouding the heart orifice. Treatment should focus on warming yáng and disinhibiting water and unblocking yáng and transforming rheum. For this, I used a modification of Zhen Wu Tang plus Wu Ling San: Fu Zi 10g, Bai Shao 10g, Gui Zhi 10g, Zhu Ling 10g, Ze Xie 10g, Bai Zhu 15g, Fu Ling 30g, Sheng Jiang 3 slices. (Five packets)

After taking the third packet, the patient suddenly began sweating from his chest and back, his urine was disinhibited, and his dizziness was partially relieved. After five packets, all symptoms were partially resolved. I then prescribed another ten packets. During the course of treatment, the patient had one small seizure and still felt slightly fatigued. I pivoted to a small dose Chun Ze Tang[10] plus Zhen Wu Tang and after taking this formula for three months, he completely recovered. Upon follow-up six years later, he reported never having a relapse.

CLINICAL INSIGHT

The patient's gaunt build, pallid complexion, spontaneous sweating, and thin, rigid-tight abdominal muscles correspond to a Gui Zhi Tang formula pattern. The back cold, substernal palpitation, lower limb edema, and inhibited urine are classic symptoms of a Wu Ling San pattern. Finally, the cold limbs, abdominal pain, dizziness, palpitations, and convulsions were all symptomatic of a Zhen Wu Tang formula pattern. The pulse and tongue were all consistent with a phlegm pattern, so I prescribed Wu Ling San plus Zhen Wu Tang. Later on, the pathogen was dispersed, but the upright qì was vacuous, so I added Dang Shen and pivoted to a smaller dose to complete his recovery. In this case, if I had just treated based on disease etiology and hadn't employed detailed formula pattern identification and herb pattern identification, I couldn't have achieved this result.

---

[10] Wu Ling San plus Ren Shen.

Obesity Treated with Modified Ban Xia Xie Xin Tang (Damp and phlegm congestion type)

MR. LIN, 40 YEARS (LABORER) (168CM, 83KG)

FIRST VISIT: September 20th, 1995

HISTORY: The patient was previously diagnosed with "obesity" and "hyperlipidemia" and had undergone ten months of treatment with Chinese medicine "weight-loss" herbs with little effect. In recent months, he seemed to be gaining weight by the day and was now up to 93kg.

CURRENT: He complains of a feeling of tightness and distention throughout his body, fatigue, desire to sleep, moistness and bitterness of the mouth with copious saliva, frequent eructation and nausea, large appetite, soft stools, borborygmus, and flatulence.

PULSE: Moderate

TONGUE: Pale with a greasy, white coating and congealed spittle.

ABDOMINAL PALPATION: Substernal hard glomus that is slightly uncomfortable upon pressing, the abdomen is large, distended, and soft to the touch.

DIAGNOSIS: This is tàiyīn disease with phlegm and dampness lodged within leading to obstruction of the upbearing and downbearing of the spleen and stomach and dysfunction of the spleen's ability to govern the four limbs. Treatment should focus on harmonizing and regulating the stomach and spleen using acrid opening and bitter descending herbs.

FORMULA: Modified Ban Xia Xie Xin Tang: Ban Xia 20g, Huang Qin 10g, Dang Shen 10g, Gan Jiang 10g, He Ye 10g, Huang Lian 3g, Zhi Gan Cao 3g, Shan Zha 30g. (Fifteen packets, one per day)

After the first course of herbs, the patient lost 3.5kg and reported increased energy, less congestion and discomfort in the stomach, decreased nausea, and that his stools were now formed. I prescribed another fifteen packets of the same formula with slight modifications. After the second course of herbs, he lost another 4kg, his substernal hard glomus improved, and he looked noticeably skinnier. I advised him to continue taking the formula in place of tea throughout the day, sipping slowly. After taking the formula in this way for another two months, his weight dropped to 75kg, his lipid panel noticeably improved, and was close to being within normal range. Upon follow-up two years later, he said his lipid panel was back to normal.

CLINICAL INSIGHT

In Chinese medicine, obesity is often believed to be the result of phlegm-damp and qì vacuity. As such, it is not difficult to diagnose the problem, but the key is to choose the correct herbs and formula. This patient had a pale tongue with a greasy, white coating with congealed spittle. This is a classic Ban Xia and Gan Jiang tongue presentation. The substernal hard glomus corresponded to a Ban Xia Xie Xin Tang pattern, and this was confirmed by the patient's "nausea, borborygmus, sloppy stool, and glomus" corresponding to the *Golden Cabinet* line: "When there is vomiting, borborygmus, and substernal glomus, Ban Xia Xie Xin Tang is indicated." I added He Ye and Shan Zha because they are specially indicated in obesity.

Cystic Hyperplasia of the Breast
(Mammary aggregation phlegm node)
Treated with Modified Xiao Chai Hu Tang
plus Xiao Xian Xiong Tang

Ms. LIU, 30 YEARS (CADRE)

FIRST VISIT: September 23rd, 1993

HISTORY: The patient related that throughout her five years of marriage to her husband, they had frequent disagreements and would often get into fights. Gradually, she began to develop cysts in both breasts that would often throb with stabbing pain. Before her period, the cysts would throb with a particularly distended, burning pain.

CURRENT: The patient is currently on her period and all symptoms are exacerbated as a result. Goose egg-like cysts can be palpated in both breasts, two on the left and one on the right. They are soft, moveable, and touch elicits pain. She complains of bitterness in the mouth, dry throat, dizziness, and dreamful sleep. Additionally, she reports bleeding from her gums when rinsing her mouth in the morning, occasionally feeling nauseous, distended pain in her stomach, and constipation.

PULSE: Wiry, slippery, and forceful

TONGUE: dark, pale red with a yellow sticky coat.

ABDOMINAL PALPATION: Discomfort upon pressing below rib-side, knocking-pain at the right ribs[11], glomus and distention from sub-sternum to above the navel with obvious pain upon pressing.

DIAGNOSIS: This is a shàoyáng yángmíng pattern with liver stagnation and phlegm heat-bind.

FORMULA: Modified Xiao Chai Hu Tang plus Xiao Xian Xiong Tang: Chai Hu 10g, Ban Xia 10g, Zhe Bei Mu 10g, Huang Qin 6g, Jie Geng 6g, Zhi Ke 6g, Huang Lian 3g, Gua Lou 20g, Xia Ku Cao 20g, Sheng Mu Li 20g, Xuan Shen 15g. (Five packets)

After her first course of herbs, the pain and distention in her breasts reduced considerably. When her period came, I added Yi Mu Cao 15g and Tao Ren 10g and prescribed another 5 packets. After taking the herbs, all symptoms continued to improve. Once her period ended, I reverted to the first formula, prescribing another fifteen packets after which the cysts noticeably shrunk. I then pivoted to a smaller dosage of the same formula and after forty packets, the cysts completely disappeared, and her abdominal presentation returned to normal. On a follow-up two years later, the cysts had not reappeared.

Clinical Insight

Breast pathologies are primarily related to shàoyáng and yángmíng. Her main symptoms of bitterness in the mouth, dry throat, dizziness, chest and rib-side fullness and discomfort, nausea, and wiry pulse correspond exactly to the shàoyáng Xiao Chai Hu Tang pattern. Her substernal glomus, fullness and pain upon pressing, and slippery pulse are indicative of a yángmíng phlegm-heat Xiao Xian Xiong Tang pattern. Breast cysts are called "mammary aggregating phlegm nodes" in Chinese medicine.

---

[11] This is a method Dr. Lou developed for testing for shàoyáng disease. He places his left hand on the rib-side and knocks on the left hand with his fisted right hand. Any discomfort indicates a shàoyáng pathology.

In this case, I combined Chai Xian Tang with Xiao Ying Wan (消瘿丸)[12] to fit both the pattern and the disease—Xia Ku Cao, Xuan Shen, and Zhe Bei Mu transform phlegm and undo binds—this combination of formula pattern identification and disease-targeted herbs yields an even faster and more effective result.

---

[12] There are several versions of this formula. Most consist of Xia Ku Cao, Zhe Bei Mu, Xuan Shen, Mu Li, Kun Bu and Hai Zao.

Synovitis Treated with Gui Zhi Tang Jia Fu Zi, Bai Zhu

FEMALE, 18 YEARS

FIRST VISIT: October 11th, 2002

The patient is a student studying abroad in France. One year ago, she developed edema and pain in both knees after a sports-related injury. She was diagnosed with synovitis and treated according to standard protocol but continued to experience frequent edema and pain. She had also gotten acupuncture and wet cupping for half a year in France, but this had been ineffective. Eventually, she decided to withdraw from school and come back to China to seek treatment.

The patient is of average height and has a robust build. She complains of pain, weakness, and aversion to cold in both knees that is present not only when walking, but also when at rest. Additionally, she reports scant, dark menses with severe period pain, and normal BMs. She claims to be afraid of needles due to a course of unsuccessful acupuncture treatments.

Based upon the cold, edematous, painful, and weak nature of her knee pathology, I prescribed Gui Zhi Tang Jia Fu Zi, Bai Zhu: Gui Zhi 10g, Bai Shao 10g, Gan Cao 5g, Sheng Jiang 5 slices, Da Zao 3 pieces, Fu Zi 10g, Bai Zhu 10g. (Seven packets)

After one week of herbs, the patient returned on October 18th and reported that there was no change in symptoms. After carefully considering her condition, I concluded that there was no problem with my diagnosis and asked her to be patient and continue taking the herbs. I then prescribed another fifteen packets of the above formula. From

October 11th to November 6th, she took herbs continuously, but there was no noticeable improvement of symptoms, and she began to lose confidence in my treatment. I conjectured that her painful period could be due to blood stagnation, so I added Gui Zhi Fu Ling Wan to the original formula and gave another fifteen packets.

On November 22nd, the patient returned to my clinic and reported that this course of herbs had been quite effective. The pain and edema in her knees had diminished and she could walk more comfortably. Her period pain had also lessened and the menstrual flow was voluminous, but there were still clots and the color was still dark. I prescribed another fifteen packets of the same formula and advised her to moxa EX-LE5 on both knees.

After another month of treatment, she made a complete recovery and happily returned to France to continue her studies. A year later, she returned to my clinic to thank me and she told me about her experience using moxa for over 6 months in great detail. She said that she would moxa EX-LE5 with stick moxa every day and had even accidentally burned herself quite a few times in the process. Yet, even if the burns blistered and ulcerated, she was determined not to miss a day of moxa and would just avoid the lesions.

CLINICAL INSIGHT

Gui Zhi Tang Jia Fu Zi, Bai Zhu is a very effective formula for treating arthritis and spinal pathologies in patients with weaker constitutions. When combined with acupuncture, the effect is even more rapid and pronounced.

The folk jīngfāng researcher Fei Wei-guang asserts that Gui Zhi Tangjia Fu Zi, Bai Zhu can treat neuralgia. His own experience with this formula is worth noting:

During the early seventies, Fei developed severe back pain after bending down to pick up his four-year-old daughter. After having one of his children lightly pound on the affected area, the pain not only failed to decrease, it actually became even worse. Treatment with electr0-acu-puncture relieved the pain while lying down, but as soon as he got up and started walking, the pain immediately returned, and he had to be carried home by a friend. He prescribed himself Gui Zhi Tang Jia Fu Zi, Bai Zhu based on his "spontaneous sweating constitution". After three packets, the pain had noticeably diminished and after another 3 packets the pain was completely resolved.

Pyogenic Arthritis of the Hip Joint
Treated with Modified Da Qing Long Tang
plus Tao He Cheng Qi Tang

MR. ZHANG, 14 YEARS

FIRST VISIT: April 6th, 1988

HISTORY: While playing with some classmates, Mr. Zhang suffered a contusion in his lower back and would often feel some discomfort in his left lower back. Then, two weeks ago, he got caught in a storm and came back home soaking wet. The next day he developed aversion to cold, high fever, back pain, and full-body pain. After taking antipyretic medication, he began to shiver, but the fever did not abate. Additionally, he began feeling severe pain and distention in left hip joint and was unable to walk. After several blood and imaging tests, he was diagnosed with pyogenic arthritis of the hip joint and herniated intervertebral disc. He was prescribed antibiotics and traction therapy, but after two weeks he still had a low fever and the pain in his hip joint had not diminished.

CURRENT: The patient has a thin build and a pallid complexion; he is fatigued and seems to be in a lot of pain. He complains of aversion to wind and cold, heat effusion with no sweating, headache, and joint and body pain. He has distention and pain in the left hip joint and the area around the joint is red, edematous, warm to the touch, and averse to touch. The pain is worse when walking and standing. He also complains of thirst, poor appetite, constipation, turbid, yellow, malodorous urine, poor sleep quality, and agitation.

TONGUE: Dark red with a white, greasy coating

PULSE: Floating, tight, and rapid

ABDOMINAL PALPATION: Pain in the left lower abdomen that extends to the inguinal area and is exacerbated upon pressing. Deep palpation reveals a soft, ropy bind.

DIAGNOSIS: This is tàiyáng-yángmíng combination disease with wind, cold, and damp congesting in the joint and transforming into heat. Treatment should focus on releasing the exterior, dispersing cold, removing damp, clearing heat, and quickening the blood.

FORMULA: Modified Da Qing Long Tang plus Tao He Cheng Qi Tang: Ma Huang, Gui Zhi, Fang Feng, Xing Ren, Tao Ren, Su Ye all 10g, Sheng Can Cao, Cang Zhu, Sheng Da Huang all 5g, Sheng Shi Gao 50g. (Three packets)

After taking the herbs, the patient had a light sweat, urine and bowel movements increased, and all symptoms were diminished. I added 10g each of Zhi Mu, Chi Shao, Fu Zi, and five slices of Sheng Jiang to make a combination of Da Qing Long Tang plus Tao He Cheng Qi Tang plus Gui Zhi Shao Yao Zhi Mu Tang and prescribed five packets.

After that course of herbs, the patient's temperature returned to normal and the redness, edema, heat, and pain in the hip joint reduced by 50–60%. I prescribed five packets of the same formula again, reducing Ma Huang to 5g and bled and cupped at spider veins over painful areas on the left hip joint.

By the fourth visit, the patient reported the pain in his hip joint had reduced by 80–90%, he could walk without discomfort and all other symptoms were resolved. However, he still had some pain in the waist upon bending at the hip. I made some modifications to the above formula, bled and cupped BL40, and did some bonesetting manipulations to correct subluxations in the lumbar vertebrae. After another two weeks of herbs, bloodletting, and manipulations, all pain subsided. The pain never returned in ten years of follow-up.

CLINICAL INSIGHT

According to master physician Yue Mei-zhong, formula pattern identification and herbal pattern identification are characterized by, "Investigating the symptom and sign presentation while rarely discussing the pathological mechanism and prescribing formulas without reference to the nature of individual herbs prescribed." *Kampo* practitioner Dōmei Yakazu (矢数道明) stated: "Kampo medicine is distinguished by its focus on treating based on pattern. As such it can be called 'symptom and pattern medicine', 'formula pattern correspondence medicine' or even 'formula medicine'. The diagnosis of symptomatology is linked directly to the formula. The diagnosis is the treatment and thus the pattern is the formula." I learned two things from this case:

This patient's sign and symptom presentation closely corresponded to the *Treatise on Cold Damage* line: "In tàiyáng windstrike disease, when there is a floating tight pulse, heat effusion, aversion to cold, body pain, lack of sweating, and agitation, Da Qing Long Tang is indicated." This line reflects the relation of this formula's pattern diagnosis to symptomology, pathology, herbal pharmacology, and theory of treatment.

Abdominal palpation is an extremely important aspect of formula pattern identification. Abdominal diagnosis saw early development in the *Yellow Emperor's Inner Canon* and *The Classic of Difficulties* and was extensively elaborated in the *Treatise on Cold Damage*. *Kampo* physician Yumoto Kyūshin (湯本求真) had this to say about abdominal diagnosis: "The abdomen is the source of life itself and is thus at the root of all disease. As such, abdominal palpation is an indispensable aspect of diagnosis." (*Imperial Han Medicine*) The tight bind extending from the patient's lower left abdomen to the left inguinal area was a classic Tao He Cheng Qi Tang abdominal presentation.

Geriatric Prostatic Hyperplasia
Treated with Modified Shen Qi Wan
(Debilitation of the life gate fire type)

MR. HUANG, 70 YEARS

FIRST VISIT: October 15th, 1992

HISTORY: The patient has suffered from benign prostatic hyperplasia for twelve years.

CURRENT: The patient has a tall and robust frame, and his complexion is pallid and edematous. He complains of frequent, scant, incomplete urination, incontinence, and frequent nocturnal urination, all of which has caused him no small amount of distress. He additionally complains of cold pain in his lower back, and coldness and discomfort in his lower abdomen. He has a normal appetite and normal bowel movements.

TONGUE: Pale red with a greasy coating restricted to the root

PULSE: Sunken, thin, and weak

ABDOMINAL PALPATION: Tension and rigidity in lower left and right abdomen

Diagnosis and Treatment: This is geriatric kidney qì vacuity and life gate fire debilitation leading to dribbling urinary block. Treatment should focus on supplementing qì, warming yáng, nourishing the kidney, and supplementing yīn.

FORMULA: Shen Qi Wan plus Dan Zhu Ye, Shi Chang Pu (Six packets)

After taking the herbs, the frequent urination improved, but all other symptoms remained unresolved. I continued prescribing another thirty packets of the same formula with slight modifications, after which the incontinence completely resolved and other symptoms improved. I then pivoted to Jin Gui Shen Qi Wan in pill form 10g twice daily. After three months, all symptoms resolved.

Acute Epididymitis Treated with Modified Long Dan Xie Gan Tang

Mr. Zhang, 40 years (farmer)

FIRST VISIT: May 10th, 1990

HISTORY: One month ago, the patient developed a fever, full-body pain and soreness, strain, distention and swelling of the left testicle with pain radiating to the inguinal area, and the left lower back, which impaired movement. He sought treatment at a hospital emergency room and was diagnosed with acute epididymitis. After a round of antibiotics, the fever partially abated, but the pain was still present, he couldn't stand up straight, was constipated, his urine was scant, and urination was painful. After 28 days of in-patient treatment at the hospital, his physician concluded that conservative treatment was proving ineffective and surgery to remove the left testicle after performing incision and drainage would be necessary. The patient did not consent to surgery and snuck out of the hospital to seek treatment from me.

CURRENT: The patient's left scrotum is red, edematous, indurated, shiny, and painful to the touch. The testicles, epididymis, and spermatic cord are all swollen and there are adhesions between the visceral and parietal layers of the tunica vaginalis. Knocking pain is present on the left lower back.

TONGUE: Dark red with a yellow, greasy, thick coating

PULSE: Wiry and rapid

125

DIAGNOSIS: This is a case of liver and gall bladder replete heat with damp heat downpouring and obstructing the liver network vessel.

I first used a three-edged needle to let blood at LR1, LR2, and LR3. The blood was dark purple and black, and after bleeding the patient noted a noticeable abatement of pain. I then prescribed two packets of Long Dan Xie Gan Tang plus Dan Shen, Tao Ren, and Da Huang and told him to cease all western medical treatment.

SECOND VISIT: May 12th

After taking the medicine, the patient had three bowel movements, the pain and distention in his scrotum was noticeably reduced, and he reported partial relief of his back pain. The scrotum was still slightly indurated upon palpation, the greasy yellow coating had slightly receded, and the pulse was wiry and rapid. I decided to use the same treatment method with slight modifications.

I first bled at left BL18, BL40, and LR3 and prescribed five packets of Long Dan Xie Gan Tang plus Ju He, Tao Ren, and Yi Ren.

THIRD VISIT: May 18th

The scrotum swelling and distention was reduced but the testicles and epididymis were still swollen, and the spermatic cord was still indurated and swollen. I bled at LR1, LR2, and SP10—the blood was lighter in color and lower in volume than the two previous times. I then prescribed San Miao Wan plus Dan Shen, Tao Ren, and Dang Gui to clear and transform lower jiao damp heat, unblock network vessels, and transform blood stasis.

FOURTH VISIT: June 3rd

Apart from some lingering induration of the spermatic cord, all other symptoms and signs had resolved.

PULSE: Wiry and thin

TONGUE: Still slightly dark red with a thin coating

ACUPUNCTURE PROTOCOL: BL18 (bilateral), BL19 (bilateral), SP10 (bilateral)

I didn't prescribe herbs and told the patient to report back if there was any lingering discomfort. Upon follow-up on July 5th, the patient informed me that he had made a full recovery. He was able to go back to work and felt as healthy as prior to the infection. Upon follow-up a year later, the patient informed me he had never had any relapse of symptoms, although he noticed that his left testicle was now slightly smaller than the right.

CLINICAL INSIGHT

Epididymitis, known as "welling-abscess of the testicle" (zǐyōng, 子癰) in Chinese, is often due to damp heat downpouring into the Juéyīn network vessel leading to qì stagnation and blood stasis. Treatment consists of bloodletting along the liver channel and Long Dan Xie Gan Tang plus blood-quickening and stasis-transforming herbs. I selected SP10 because it can quicken the blood, fortify the spleen, and transform dampness. In this case, the patient was treated with Western medicine for over a month with poor results. The doctor was preparing to perform surgery, but the patient switched to Chinese medicine and his condition resolved rapidly. This was a truly amazing result. From this case, we can also see how powerful bloodletting is as a healing modality.

The patient was a relative of mine, and so I've been able to follow-up with him often over the years. Though he's since had other illnesses, he has never developed epididymitis again.

Painful Suppurative Peri-anal Ulcers after Anul Fistula Surgery Treated with Gan Cao Xie Xin Tang plus Ling Gui Zao Gan Tang

Ms. C, 18 YEARS (155CM, 42KG)

FIRST VISIT: August 7th, 2015

CC: Recurrent painful suppurative ulcers around the anus for five years subsequent to anal fistula surgery

HISTORY: The patient is currently a student and has been prescribed steroids for her condition, but she still frequently develops peri-anal suppurative ulcers and suffers from abdominal pain. She was found to have terminal ileus erosion, an ileocecal valve ulcer, and colon aphthous ulcers and was eventually diagnosed with Crohn's Disease. In addition, blood tests and exams revealed a complicated picture: She had pelvic effusion, elevated proteinuria and leukocyturia, chronic atrophic gastritis with erosion, bile reflux gastritis, occult blood in the stool, jejunal mucosa follicular hyperplasia, small intestine multi-segment inflammation, and other findings which were all consistent with a diagnosis of Crohn's disease.

CURRENT: The patient is of average height but has an anemic complexion and appears emaciated and undernourished. She complains of occasional low fever, canker sores, dry mouth, halitosis, occasional abdominal pain, abdominal distention, diarrhea, sticky and malodorous stools passed four to five times per day, peri-anal distention, pain, heat and itchiness, yellow, malodorous, frequent, scant urine, borborygmus, and scant menses. She claims to have a good appetite.

PULSE: Wiry and rapid.

TONGUE: red with thin coating.

ABDOMINAL PALPATION: Average springiness, substernal glomus, periumbilical tightness, and aversion to touch.

DIAGNOSIS: Gan Cao Xie Xin Tang and Bao He Wan pattern.

I first prescribed Bao He Wan:

Shan Zha 10g, Shen Qu 10g, Ban Xia 10g, Fu Ling 15g, Chen Pi 10g, Lian Qiao 5g, Lai Fu Zi 10g. (Seven packets, one per day)

SECOND VISIT: August 15th

The patient reported that after taking the formula for four days, she passed a large amount of sticky, malodorous stool and exudate, after which her abdominal distention was reduced. All other symptoms, however, were still present. Upon palpation, I noticed that the periumbilical tightness was gone, but there was still some aversion to pressing. Upon deep palpation below the navel, I noted her abdominal aorta had a bounding, strong pulse.

DIAGNOSIS: Gan Cao Xie Xin Tang plus Ling Gui Zao Gan Tang pattern

Gan Cao 15g, Huang Qin 10g, Gan Jiang 10g, Ban Xia 10g, Dang Shen 10g, Huang Lian 5g, Da Zao 6g, Fu Ling 20g, Gui Zhi 10g. (Fifteen packets, one packet per day. After taking five packets, rest one day.)

THIRD VISIT: September 5ᵗʰ

The patient's temperature returned to normal, canker sores reduced in size and number, diarrhea abated, borborygmus improved, peri-anal discomfort improved, and urination frequency decreased. Her mood seemed improved, and she had grown more confident in my treatment. However, she still complained of abdominal pain, distention, sticky and malodorous stools 1–2 times per day, dry mouth, halitosis, and delayed menses.

PULSE: Wiry

TONGUE: Red with little coating

ABDOMINAL PALPATION: Moderate springiness, substernal hard glomus.

FORMULA:Gan Cao 15g, Huang Qin 10g, Gan Jiang 6g, Ban Xia 10g, Dang Shen 15g, Huang Lian 5g, Da Zao 10 pieces, Fu Ling 20g, Gui Zhi 10g. (Fifteen packets, one packet per day. After five packets, rest one day.)

SEPTEMBER 24ᵗʰ: On the fifth day of her period, she reports scant menses. Her canker sores have completely resolved, diarrhea resolved, borborygmus was reduced, frequent urination resolved, and only had occasional abdominal pain and distention. She still complained of bitterness in the mouth, halitosis, sloppy, and malodorous, unformed stools 1–2 times per day.

PULSE: wiry

TONGUE: Red with little coating

ABDOMINAL PALPATION: Moderate springiness, substernal hard glomus, palpitations on and below navel.

FORMULA: Same as above, (Fifteen packets, one packet per day. After five packets, rest one day.

After three months of treatment using this basic formula, her stools returned to normal, all blood tests returned to within normal range, her weight increased, and her menstrual cycle was regulated.

Clinical Insight

This patient had a particularly complicated presentation. In my clinical process, I was primarily guided by the finding of "periumbilical tension and pain upon pressing", which I believe to be a Bao He Wan abdominal finding. As such, I first prescribed a week of Bao He Wan. After four packets, she passed a large amount of sticky, malodorous stool and exudate, after which her abdominal distention was reduced. This result paved the way for the rest of the treatment.

Through many years of practice, I found that periumbilical tension and pain upon pressing are indicative of a Bao He Wan pattern. I often get surprisingly good results using this abdominal pattern, especially in children. This pattern has to be differentiated from Gui Zhi Fu Ling Wan and other blood stasis patterns that also present with periumbilical pain upon pressing.

The patient's canker sores, dry mouth, halitosis, occasional abdominal pain, abdominal distention, diarrhea, sticky and malodorous stools, yellow and malodorous urine, frequent and scant urination, and borborygmus are all suggestive of a Xie Xin Tang pattern, but I was only able to confirm that it was specifically a Gan Cao Xie Xin Tang pattern after observing the moderate abdominal springiness and substernal hard glomus. This demonstrates the decisive role abdominal diagnosis plays in jīngfāng treatment.

When a patient presents with palpitations on and below the navel and moderate abdominal springiness, this is often suggestive of a Ling Gui Wu Wei Gan Cao Tang or Ling Gui Zao Gan Tang pattern. If there is weak abdominal springiness, then Dang Gui Shao Yao San, Ba Zhen Tang, and Shen Qi Wan should be considered.

However, how does one determine what qualifies as moderate abdominal springiness as opposed to strong or weak springiness? This is something that has to be felt and intuited, it can't be quantified. This is a kind of knowledge that develops through practice. Indeed, much of the knowledge encapsulated in the jīngfāng system is of this type. In the course of study, apart from mastering the objective knowledge presented in the texts, one must also acquire an experiential knowledge through clinical practice.

Impetigo Treated with Gui Zhi Jia Huang Qi Tang

6 YEARS, FEMALE

The patient began developing impetigo lesions on her forearm, back, and abdomen six months ago. The lesions steadily grew in size and worsened in severity despite continuous treatment.

FIRST VISIT: January 7th, 2012

The patient has light skin, an endomorphic build, and a ruddy complexion. Her parents informed me that she easily catches colds and sweats profusely in the summer. The colds typically manifest with heat effusion, headache, phlegmy cough and are often protracted. Based upon the clinical experience of Ōtsuka Keisetsu, I prescribed Gui Zhi Jia Huang Qi Tang.

After a week of herbs the impetigo lesions on her arm and back reduced by half. After another two weeks of herbs, her condition continued to improve but was still not completely stable. Overall, it seemed that treatment was headed in the right direction.

After another week of the same formula, new lesions stopped forming and the lesions on her abdomen were gradually receding. I continued using the same formula combined with Yu Ping Feng San: Huang Qi 10g, Gui Zhi 5g, Bai Shao 5g, Gan Cao 3g, Sheng Jiang 2 slices, Da Zao 2 pieces, Bai Zhu 5g, Fang Feng 5g. (Seven packets)

After this course of herbs, the condition completely resolved. Six months later, she had a relapse that was again resolved with one week of Gui Zhi j Huang Qi Tang. Since then, there have been no relapses.

In *Imperial Medicine*, Ōtsuka states that Huang Qi is indicated for patients with weak constitutions when water toxins collect in the skin and lead to dermatological conditions due to poor circulation and nourishment of the skin. He describes it as a supplementing, sweat-checking, and urine disinhibiting herb. I have treated many cases of pediatric impetigo using this interpretation of the Gui Zhi Jia Huang Qi Tang formula pattern.

CLINICAL INSIGHT

There are guiding principles in clinical Chinese medicine, but it is still possible for two different physicians to come to completely different diagnoses regarding the same patient. That being said, some diagnostic systems are better than others.

There are two approaches to treatment in Chinese medicine: the disease-targeted approach and the pattern-targeted approach, the latter being concerned with the patient's pathological manifestation of the body's response to illness. Jīngfāng medicine demands the physician to take a bird's-eye view of the patient's entire physiological function in the context of the body's response to the pathogen. The Hungarian Marxist philosopher György Lukács once stated: "In the case of systemic problems, we should not expect to resolve them via changes to various parts of the whole in isolation." Jīngfāng medicine's emphasis on formula pattern and constitutional diagnosis is a reflection of its focus on the holistic response of the body in its struggle against the pathogen. This approach can help compensate for the deficiencies of the disease-targeted specialist medicine of today.

Festering, Painful Burn Wound on the Calf Treated with Gui Zhi Tang

20 YEARS, MALE

The patient sustained a burn on the left calf one month ago after being scorched by the exhaust pipe on his motorbike during an accident. The burn began to fester and ulcerate, but despite western medical treatment, he saw no improvement in his condition and the lesion was still extremely painful.

FIRST VISIT: August 15th, 1998

The patient was helped into my clinic by family.

The patient has an average build, slightly dark complexion and a knitted brow, and grimace-like expression due to the pain of the lesion. The lesion is about 50 cm², has a foul odor and is extremely painful. The patient complains of headache, agitated heat (37.5°C), aversion to wind, sweating, dry mouth with no desire to drink, insomnia (due to pain), and weight loss (4kg in two weeks). Appetite is normal, urine is normal, and he reports slight constipation.

PULSE: Rapid

TONGUE: Pale red, white coating.

Surveying his symptoms, the heat effusion, headache, aversion to wind, and sweating were all consistent with a Gui Zhi Tang pattern. I reasoned that the constipation might not be related to the current pathology as he explained it was a long-standing problem. As such, I prescribed Gui Zhi Tang and instructed him to take it according to the *Treatise on Cold Damage* instructions (After drinking the herbs, eat some warm congee, and then cover yourself with a blanket. If you get a light sweat and the symptoms resolve, then there is no need to take the second dose. If there is no sweat, take another dose and follow the same instructions.)

SECOND VISIT: August 18ᵗʰ

The patient reported that after taking the herbs, he began to sweat much more. His aversion to wind, headache, and calf pain all diminished, the wound began to heal, and the fever abated. Based upon the above symptoms, I pivoted to Yu Ping Feng San plus Dang Gui. In a follow-up call two months later, the patient reported that the wound had steadily healed and all that was left now was a faint scar.

CLINICAL INSIGHT

This was the first burn wound I ever treated. As is quite clear, I didn't treat this patient based on the pathomechanism, but rather by using formula pattern correspondence. The clinical efficacy of this approach demonstrates that it is worthy of deep research and study. There are those who believe formula pattern diagnosis is a low or beginner level of diagnosis and treatment, but nothing could be further from the truth. A pathomechanism-based form of treatment might involve the following analysis of this case: The high heat of the burn created a heat toxin to invade via the skin leading to qì and blood stasis and eventually caused the skin to fester. The agitated heat, protracted pain, constipation, and rapid pulse also indicate qì and blood stasis as well as heat toxin invading the construction and blood layers. Based upon this analysis, in addition to using a plaster on the wound, Huang Lian Jie Du Tang plus Xi Jiao Di Huang Tang would be the first-choice formula to clear heat, drain fire, and cool and quicken the blood. This analysis and treatment approach could not be more at odds with a Gui Zhi Tang diagnosis. Why is it that two different diagnostic systems could arrive at such different conclusions when faced with the very same patient? This is a question worth pondering.

Formula pattern diagnosis is the core component of jīngfāng medicine. For the jīngfāng practitioner, learning how to identify the key symptoms that point to a particular formula pattern correspondence is an important and foundational skill. Perfecting this foundational skill requires that one applies themselves in a concerted fashion to the practice of formula pattern diagnosis.

The famous Qing dynasty physician Xu Lingtai (徐靈台) stated: "In the past, I also believed that the *Treatise on Cold Damage* might have been compiled incorrectly and was in need of reordering, but after thirty years of practice, I finally came to a realization and began thinking of the *Treatise* in terms of formulas as opposed to conformations (經, sometimes called channels). For, formulas have a set way in which they treat disease, but diseases are protean and ever-changing in nature. Once one grasps what each formula treats, the prescription can be adjusted based upon the myriad changes by which diseases manifest.

Another physician who commented on the proper approach to jīngfāng medicine was Yu Jiayan (喻嘉言), a famous physician who died ten years before Xu Lingtai was born and wrote *Notes on My Judgment* (寓意草) and *Precepts for Physicians* (醫門法律) among other books. Yu was a skilled jīngfāng clinician, but he had a different approach from Xu Lingtai. Yu emphasized that the key to treatment in jīngfāng was to identify the main disease. Thus, in *Notes on My Judgment*, he has cases in which he uses Li Zhong Tang to treat the *diseases* of malaria, cholera, and glomus, while using Tao He Cheng Qi Tang plus Fu Zi, Rou Gui to treat paralysis of the lower limbs. He stated, "One must first determine the disease before proceeding with treatment and prescribing herbs" and "Once the disease and channel have been identified, then prescribe herbs based upon the disease. For the thousand different diseases, there are a thousand different herbal formulas." Sit with these ideas and ponder them over: whose theory do you think is best?

Recurrent Urticaria Treated with
Gui Zhi Er Yue Bi Yi Tang

MIDDLE-AGED, FEMALE

HISTORY: The patient has suffered from urticaria for three years. Her flares were well controlled with Chinese medicine, but she became frustrated by their frequent recurrence. After a recent trip, she had another flare and despite taking Chinese medicine and using herbal plasters, the urticaria did not resolve, so she sought me out for treatment.

FIRST VISIT: January 5th, 2013

The patient has a pallid, anemic complexion. The urticaria hives are mainly concentrated on her arms, legs, lower back, and abdomen. The hives are about the size of a matchstick head, pale red, raised, and extremely itchy. She additionally complains of aversion to wind, thirst, agitation, redness of the face, agitation and heat, and sweating. Her last period was one week ago for which she reports scant volume and dark color. Her urine, BMs, and appetite are normal.

PULSE: Floating and tight

TONGUE: Pale red with a thin white coating.

Based upon these symptoms, I prescribed three packets of Gui Zhi Er Yue Bi Yi Tang.

Gui Zhi 10g, Bai Shao 10g, Sheng Jiang 3 slices, Da Zao 3 pieces, Gan Cao 5g, Sheng Ma Huang 5g, Xing Ren 10g, Sheng Shi Gao 15g (Take the herbs warm and lie down and cover with a blanket to promote a light sweat.)

After taking the first packet, the patient called saying the hives had gotten worse and asked if she should continue. I thought that this was probably a mìnxuàn reaction and instructed her to continue. Before even taking the second dose of her third packet, the hives completely disappeared. She had never seen the hives abate that quickly in three years of suffering from urticaria.

SECOND VISIT: January 9th, 2013

The patient complained of bitterness of the mouth, yellow urine, vertigo, and had a wiry and thin pulse.

FORMULA: Xiao Chai Hu Tang plus Fang Feng, Jing Jie (Five packets)

On follow-up one year later, she reported never having another recurrence.

CLINICAL INSIGHT

Gui Zhi Er Yue Bi Yi Tang is a modification of Da Qing Long Tang. Da Qing Long Tang strongly promotes sweating and clears interior heat. Gui Zhi Er Yue Bi Yi Tang is an acrid, cooling formula that promotes a light sweat—it is targeted at relatively superficial disease and moderate symptoms. Professor Li Tongxian (李同宪) believes that both Gui Zhi Er Yue Bi Yi Tang and Da Qing Long Tang treat a disease state in transition from the exterior to the interior. Gui Zhi Er Yue Bi Yi Tang treats the transition state between a Gui Zhi Tang and Bai Hu Tang pattern, while Da Qing Long Tang treats the transition state between a Ma Huang Tang and Bai Hu Tang pattern.

Line 27 of the *Treatise on Cold Damage* states: "In tàiyáng disease, when there is heat effusion and aversion to cold with more heat than cold (if the pulse is weak, this means yang is vacuous and sweating should be avoided), Gui Zhi Er Yue Bi Yi Tang can be used." The Kang Ping version of the *Treatise* omits "this means yang is vacuous". Later commentators have done a lot of research into this line, but it was perhaps a wasted effort given that this part of the line did not even exist in the Kang Ping version.

The formula pattern for Gui Zhi Er Yue Bi Yi Tang is moderate heat effusion and aversion to cold with more heat effusion than cold, and should also include agitation and vexation, redness of the face, thirst, and other heat symptoms. The itchiness of the hives in urticaria can count as a kind of "agitation and vexation".

This is a combination formula and does not appear in the Kang Zhi version of the *Treatise* or the *Essential Prescriptions*. It first surfaces in the Song Ben version of the *Treatise*. This indicates that successive versions of the *Treatise* progressed from relatively simple formulas to more complex and fully formed formulas.

In jīngfāng medicine, there are several tens of formula patterns used to address urticaria, reflecting the true and varied manifestation of this disease. As long as the formula corresponds to the pattern, the treatment will be successful. *Essentials of Kampo Medicine Dermatology Treatment* (日本漢方醫學皮膚病治療輯要) is a great clinical reference on this topic.

Shingles Treated with Xiao Xian Xiong Tang plus Da Huang

80 YEARS, MALE

The patient is tall and thin with a pallid complexion and a gaunt face. I originally treated this patient for abdominal pain subsequent to stomach cancer surgery. He related that he had suffered from dull pain in the periumbilical area of his abdomen for thirty years and that the pain had worsened after surgery. He had also had cardiac stent surgery in the past. The patient had a thin and wiry pulse, was constipated, and had paper-thin, tight abdominal muscles. I prescribed seven packets of Gui Zhi Jia Da Huang Tang, after which his abdominal pain was significantly reduced. After another seven packets, the pain completely abated. His whole family came to the clinic to tell me the good news and they were all amazed by the result.

Six months later, he returned to my clinic complaining of painful shingles on his face for five days that hadn't responded to other forms of treatment. Upon diagnosis, I found he had a symptomology consistent with a combination of Gui Zhi Jia Da Huang, Xiao Chai Hu Tang, and Xiao Xian Xiong Tang patterns. I combined the three formulas and prescribed three packets. However, after taking the herbs, there was little change in symptomology. After careful consideration, I concluded that this was a tàiyáng-shàoyáng dragover disease. The tàiyáng aspect corresponded to a Gui Zhi Tang pattern, but there were two possibilities for shàoyáng—it was either a Xiao Chai Hu Tang pattern or a Xiao Xian Xiong Tang plus Da Huang pattern. I first gave him three packets of Chai Hu Gui Zhi Tang. After taking the first packet, the night pain from the shingles significantly diminished and after three days of herbs, the pain flares completely ceased. However, he still had a Xiao Xian Xiong Tang plus Da Huang pattern, so I gave him five packets of that formula. After completing this course of herbs, all symptoms resolved.

There is an interesting postscript to this story. One year after treating the patient, his daughter came to my clinic seeking treatment and told me that her father had passed away one month ago. I felt a little bit uneasy and was worried that perhaps her father had been unsatisfied with my treatment. To my surprise, his daughter told me that before he passed, her father had said: "I suffered from abdominal pain for thirty years and never found a doctor during that time that could treat it. Who would have thought that I would end up getting better after just a few packets of Dr. Lou's herbs. If I had come across him sooner, I think I might have been able to live a few more years. The first medicine he gave me for the shingles wasn't right, it had an odd taste. But the second prescription was different—as soon as I drank it down, I started feeling more comfortable and soon after that I fell asleep. After I pass, if you girls get sick make sure to go see Dr. Lou and don't bother with Western medicine. If you see him again, make sure to tell him what I've said."

HIVD Treated with Modified
Gui Zhi Xin Jia Tang plus Wu Ling San
(Tàiyáng Type)

Mr. Zheng, 50 years

FIRST VISIT: September 20th, 1995

HISTORY: The patient has suffered from chronic, intermittent lower back pain for ten years. In recent years, symptoms have intensified—the patient complains of sinking pain in the lower left back, pain and soreness in the left gluteal region, and intermittent claudication. He was diagnosed with L4–5 HIVD and degenerative lumbar spinal stenosis via x-ray and CT scan.

CURRENT: The patient is gaunt with a pallid complexion. He complains of dull pain and numbness in his lower back and legs, inability to stand up straight, and limited bending mobility in the back. He complains of occasional aversion to wind, heat effusion, spontaneous sweating, vertigo, poor appetite, sleepiness, overproduction of saliva in the mouth, sloppy stools, scant and yellow urine, and slight edema of the lower limbs.

TONGUE: Pale red with a thin, white, moist coating.

PULSE: Sunken, moderate, and forceless

ABDOMINAL PALPATION: The abdominal wall is thin, the abdomen is flat and tight, palpitations can be felt at the navel, the lower abdomen is distended and full, and there is pain upon pressing at the lower back and coccyx.

This is a combination tàiyáng channel and bowel disease. Construction and defense are disharmonized, wind, cold, and damp have congealed and blocked the tàiyáng channel, and there is rheum congestion in the tàiyáng bowel. Modified Gui Zhi Xin Jia Tang plus Wu Ling San is indicated to harmonize defense and construction, disinhibit water and damp, and dispel wind and cold.

FORMULA: Gui Zhi 15g, Dang Shen 15g, Bai Shao 30g, Da Zao 5g, Chao Bai Zhu 10g, Fu Ling 10g, Zhu Ling 10g, Ze Xie 10g, Zhi Gan Cao 5g, Shao Ren 5g, Sheng Jiang 5 slices. (3 packets)

After taking the herbs, the patient reported increased urine volume, decreased aversion to wind and heat effusion, and improved appetite. However, there was no noticeable change in the back and leg pain. I targeted this unimproved symptom by adding 10g of Fu Zi to increase the cold dispelling and yáng warming function of the formula. After taking another five packets, the patient reported a decrease in back and leg pain, but he still had significantly limited bending mobility in the back. The above formula hit the mark, so I prescribed another five packets and performed massage and wet cupping on sensitive areas of the lower back and coccyx to assist the flow of qì and blood.

After another three weeks of using various modifications of this formula, all symptoms resolved and the tightness in his abdomen was reduced, however he still had significant weakness and tiredness in his legs upon exercise. I advised the patient to use moxa daily at DU2, GB30, and RN4 to gently warm and supplement yáng qì and restore function. After using moxa for one month, he made a complete recovery. On a follow-up four years later, the patient reported that he never had a serious relapse of pain and just felt some slight discomfort in his lower back and legs after performing heavy labor.

CLINICAL INSIGHT

The *Treatise on Cold Damage* provides a comprehensive theory of disease, and a diagnostic system based upon six-conformation diagnosis. The Qing Dynasty physician Ke Qin (柯琴) stated: "What few understand is that Zhong-jing's method can be applied to all disease—all diseases are encompassed within the six-conformation system without exception. One must seek the source of disease in terms of the six conformation system and not grasp at mere names and classifications which are the branch-tip and leaf of the disease." This is certainly also the case in the treatment of HIVD. The tàiyáng section of the *Treatise on Cold Damage* has the most detailed analysis of wind, cold, and damp impediment. Tàiyáng is the outer fencing of the body and the first to come up against wind, cold, and damp evil as it tries to infiltrate the body, inducing a holistic reaction as it passes from the channels to the bowels, and from the exterior to the interior.

This patient had a thin build, pallid complexion, aversion to cold, heat effusion, and spontaneous sweating—symptoms consistent with a Gui Zhi Tang pattern. The flat abdomen with tightness and rigidity is a Gui Zhi Xin Jia Tang abdominal pattern. After several years of lower back and leg pain, the patient had significant qì and blood vacuity. Additionally, despite having symptoms like aversion to wind, heat effusion, and spontaneous sweating, which were consistent with a tàiyáng wind-strike pattern, his pulse was sunken, moderate, and forceless, a finding consistent with the indications for Gui Zhi Xin Jia Tang: "If after sweating, there is body pain and a sunken and slow pulse, Gui Zhi Xin Jia Tang is indicated." The patient's umbilical palpitations, lower abdomen distention and fullness, inhibited urine, lower leg edema, and moist and white tongue coating were indicative of a tàiyáng Wu Ling San water amassment syndrome in which the tàiyáng channel syndrome failed to resolve and damp cold passed from the channel into the tàiyáng bowel. Because this appeared to be a tàiyáng channel-bowel combination disease, I first prescribed Gui Zhi Xin Jia Tang plus Wu Ling San to harmonize construction and defense, unblock yáng, and disinhibit water. This is known as the "unblocking yang via disinhibiting urine as opposed to warming" method. Once the condition had stabilized, I had the patient use moxa to gently warm and supplement yáng to reinforce the treatment efficacy.

HIVD Treated with Modified
Chai Hu Gui Zhi Tang plus Shen Zhuo Tang
(Shàoyáng-Tàiyáng Combination Disease Type)

Mr. Li, 35 years

FIRST VISIT: August 16th, 1992

HISTORY: The patient sustained a blunt force injury to his lower back two years ago which later caused him to develop pain and numbness in his lower back and legs. Upon physical examination, the patient was found to have levoscoliosis, L5 spinous process subluxation, pain upon pressing around the S1 spinous process, pain upon pressing at the sacroiliac joint with a ropy bind and a positive left straight leg raise test. X-ray revealed a narrowing of the L5-S1 disc with bone bridge formation. He was diagnosed with HIVD secondary to left sacroiliac joint subluxation.

CURRENT: The patient is tall, thin, and grimaces with pain. He complains of coldness, pain, heaviness, stiffness, spasming, and reduced sideways mobility in the lower back. Additionally, he reports aversion to cold, hot agitation, bitterness in the mouth, dry throat, nausea, and scant, incomplete urine.

TONGUE: Pale red with a thick, yellow, greasy, moist coating

PULSE: Sunken and wiry

DIAGNOSIS: This is a case of damp, wind, and cold lodging in tàiyáng, infiltrating from the exterior to the interior and subsequently damaging shàoyáng, leading to a two-conformation combination disease. Treatment should focus on resolving the flesh, expelling wind and cold, harmonizing shàoyáng, and eliminating dampness.

FORMULA: Chai Hu Gui Zhi Tang plus Shen Zhuo Tang: Chai Hu, Huang Qin, Gui Zhi, Bai Shao, Dang Shen, Gan Jiang, Ban Xia, Bai Zhu, Fu Ling all 10g, Gan Cao 5g, Sheng Jiang 5 slices, Da Zao 5 pieces. (Five packets)

I additionally needled GB30 on the left side.

After three packets, all symptoms improved and after five packets, the patient's left leg numbness noticeably diminished. This was clearly the right formula, so I prescribed another five packets and performed massage and acupuncture.

On his third visit, the patient reported that all symptoms had noticeably improved. I added Xi Xin to reinforce the cold dispelling and channel warming effect of the formula. After using modifications of the same formula for a month, the condition completely resolved. On a follow-up in 2000, the patient reported being in good health with no discomfort in his lower back.

Clinical Insight

I use Chai Hu formulas in HIVD based upon the idea that as a pivot, shàoyáng formulas not only prevent a situation in which "blood and qì become vacuous, the interstices open, and evil qì enters" but also mediate the qì dynamic to outthrust evils within. Chai Hu formulas can be used not only to treat Chai Hu patterns and Chai Hu constitutions, but also more broadly in dragover and combination diseases in which the pathological dynamic is in flux.

Xiao Chai Hu Tang is the primary formula for shàoyáng disease, but it can also be used in triple yáng combination disease. I diagnosed this patient as having shàoyáng-tàiyáng combination disease based upon this *Treatise and Cold Damage* line: "When there is heat effusion, slight aversion to cold, agitation and pain in the joints of the limbs, slight nausea, and substernal propping and binding, the exterior condition has not resolved, and Chai Hu Gui Zhi Tang is indicated." The urinary bladder and kidney have an exterior-interior relationship—the patient's coldness and pain in the lower back was a result of cold-damp invading the tàiyáng urinary bladder channel, a dynamic that coincides closely to the *Essential Prescriptions of the Golden Cabinet* line: "In kidney fixity disease, the body feels heavy, and the lower back is cold...Gan Jiang Ling Zhu Tang (Shen Zhuo Tang) is indicated." The treatment was effective because I understood the passage and transmutation logic of Chai Hu formulas and successfully identified a formula that corresponded to the presenting pattern.

The Shi family traumatology lineage (石氏傷科) was known for their special use of Chai Hu formulas in internal damage subsequent to external injury, but they justified this usage by saying that when "treating blood, one must invariably also treat qì, and when treating qì, one must invariably course the liver." This theory was difficult for successive generations to grasp, so this methodology never gained wider recognition.

HIVD Treated with Gui Zhi Jia Huang Qi Tang plus Wu Ling San (Tàiyīn Disease Type)

MS. JIANG, 25 YEARS

FIRST VISIT: March 20th, 1999

The patient began experiencing numbness and pain in her legs and lower back six years ago and was subsequently diagnosed with HIVD via x-ray, CT, and MRI. In the past two months, her condition has worsened.

CURRENT: The patient reports feeling soreness and weakness in her lower back and hips accompanied by spasms in the muscles of the lumbar and coccyx area. There is pain upon pressing around the L4, L5, and S1 spinous processes. She is thin and has a pallid complexion and expressive eyes. She complains of headaches, heat vexation, sweating, thirst and susceptibility to cold. She reports that she has periocular and facial edema upon waking, obstructed urine, and significant night sweats. Her period is typically delayed with dark, clotted menses, and severe pre-menstrual abdominal pain and leukorrhea.

TONGUE: Pale with a thick, white, watery coating.

PULSE: Sunken, wiry, and slippery.

ABDOMINAL PALPATION: The abdomen is flat, and the abdominal muscles are tight and rigid. Upon palpation, there is pain upon pressing at the left lower abdomen, periumbilical palpitation, and substernal splash sound.

DIAGNOSIS: This is tàiyīn impediment disease. yáng qì is stagnant, and the spleen is vacuous and congested with dampness, which has led to a breakdown of transformation.

FORMULA: Gui Zhi Jia Huang Qi Tang plus Wu Ling San: Huang Qi 30g, Gui Zhi 15g, Bai Shao 15g, Bai Zhu 15g, Fu Ling 10g, Ze Xie 10g, Zhu Ling 10g, Da Zao 3 pieces, Sheng Jiang 10 slices. (Five packets)

After taking the herbs, the patient felt a sense of warmth and comfort throughout her body. Her urinary volume increased, edema decreased, and the lower back and leg pain was slightly diminished. The formula was on target, so I prescribed another five packets. I also massaged her lumbosacral area and needled GB30.

After thirty days of various modifications of this formula, the patient's intractable disease was cured. However, upon palpation, I noticed she still had rigidity in her abdomen and pain upon pressing at the left lower abdomen. I advised her to moxa at RN6 and take Gui Zhi Fu Ling Wan in pill form. After two months, all symptoms were resolved, and her menstrual symptoms all disappeared. On a follow-up one year later, she reported being able to perform hard physical labor.

CLINICAL INSIGHT

"Observe the pulse and symptoms, identify the site of counterflow and disorder, and treat according to the pattern" is Zhong-jing's guiding principle for diagnosis and treatment. "Identify the site of counterflow and disorder" means to arrive at a diagnosis through an analysis of the mechanism. "Treat according to the pattern" means to arrive at a diagnosis via formula and herb pattern correspondence. In this case, the patient had tàiyīn impediment disease, yáng qì stagnation, and the spleen was vacuous and congested with dampness—this is a mechanism-based diagnosis. Subsequently, I then prescribed Gui Zhi Jia Huang Qi Tang plus Wu Ling San based upon a formula pattern diagnosis. The first form of diagnosis focuses on the disease's universal contradiction, whereas the latter focuses on the disease's particular contradiction—[13] only by combining these two approaches can diagnosis and treatment encapsulate the totality of the disease.

I gained two major insights regarding formula pattern diagnosis through this case: 1.) To practice formula pattern diagnosis, the practitioner must be extremely familiar with the original lines of the *Treatise on Cold Damage* and *Essential Prescriptions of the Golden Cabinet*. For instance, in this case, I recognized how the patient's lower back and hip soreness, weakness, and pain with spasms in the lower back and coccyx was similar to the *Essential Prescriptions* line "Looseness and pain of the lower back and hips with an appearance of something lodged in the skin", and thus I prescribed Gui Zhi Jia Huang Qi Tang. 2.) A patient's constitution will often lead them to be sensitive to certain substances and have a compatibility with certain herbal compounds. The 19th to 20th century *kampo* physician Mori Dōhaku (森道伯) called constitution patterns "congenital patterns". Constitutional herb pattern diagnosis, itself a subclass of herb pattern diagnosis, focuses on the clinical symptomatology that helps identify constitutional types and the corresponding herbal formulas to which they will respond favorably. For instance, this patient had a Huang Qi pattern with an underlying Gui Zhi constitution. Her pallid complexion, gaunt build, expressive eyes, spontaneous sweating, and susceptibility to contracting colds were all indicative of a Gui Zhi constitution, while her profuse sweating with swelling and heaviness in the body were indicative of a Huang Qi pattern. Because a patient's constitutional pattern is less subject to change, Gui Zhi formulas were involved in every step of this patient's treatment, from Gui Zhi Jia Huang Qi Tang, to

---

[13] Here, Dr. Lou is borrowing a concept from Marxism developed in Chairman Mao's *On Contradiction* (矛盾論). The basic idea is that concepts like "spleen vacuity" and "tàiyīn impediment disease" are generalizable across a wide array of disease processes—in this sense they represent the universal nature of the contradictory process of disease. (Contradiction, in Marxist terms is just the tension between opposites that is at the foundation of and drives all meaning, value, history etc.) By contrast, the "particularity of contradiction" is the idea that within generalizable, universal processes, one can zoom in on specific details and identify unique contradictions, or tensions and dynamics that are different from other situations. In this case, Dr. Lou is saying that formula pattern correspondence embodies the particularity of contradiction insofar as each formula pattern is specifically delineated with details of a unique symptom presentation.

Wu Ling San, to Gui Zhi Fu Ling Wan. By contrast, the patient's Huang Qi pattern was more temporary, so as soon as the pattern changed, I removed this herb.

HIVD Treated with Ma Huang Fu Zi Gan Cao Tang plus Fu Zi Tang (Shàoyīn Type)

Ms. Qian, 30 years

FIRST VISIT: September 28th, 2000

HISTORY: The patient sustained an injury to her lower back in a car accident two years ago and developed pain in her lumbosacral region that radiated to both legs. Recently, the pain has notably increased. She was diagnosed with HIVD and lumbar recess stenosis via CT and x-ray.

CURRENT: The patient has a slightly overweight build, appears fatigued and in pain, and has a sallow and dry complexion. Her lower back is rigid, painful, and immobile and the lateral portions of both legs are cold, numb, and painful. She complains of rhinorrhea, diminished sense of smell, sloppy stools, and inhibited, frequent urine.

TONGUE: Engorged, dark and pale with a thick, white, watery coating.

PULSE: Wiry, thin, weak, and slow.

ABDOMINAL PALPATION: The abdomen is overall lax and soft and gives way with pressing, but the muscle around the navel is rigid and pressing radiates pain to the back.

DIAGNOSIS: The patient has shàoyīn disease against the backdrop of a Ma Huang constitution. yáng and blood are vacuous and wind, damp, and

156

cold have lodged in the back and legs. treatment should focus on warming yáng, dispelling cold, and disinhibiting dampness.

FORMULA: Ma Huang Fu Zi Gan Cao Tang plus Fu Zi Tang: Fu Zi 10g, Bai Zhu 10g, Fu Ling 10g, Dang Shen 10g, Bai Shao 10g, Ma Huang 5g, Gan Cao 5g. (Five packets)

I also did bonesetting manipulations to correct the subluxated lumbar vertebrae and wet cupped at painful sites on the lower back and legs.

After treatment, all symptoms improved. I added Xi Xin and Dang Gui to penetrate into the yíng and blood layers and prescribed another five packets. I also massaged her upper back and lumbosacral area. After using the same method for another two weeks, the patient felt warmth return to her limbs, her edema was diminished, urine disinhibited, stools became formed, and lumbosacral and lower limb pain gradually subsided. I then pivoted to Yang He Tang for another two months, after which she made a complete recovery. On a follow-up six months later, she reported that she was now able to walk like she had before her illness.

CLINICAL INSIGHT

This patient had a Fu Zi pattern and Fu Zi pulse against the backdrop of a Ma Huang Constitution. (Ma Huang Constitution: overweight, averse to cold, dark and dry complexion, tendency to develop edema, and dry skin with no sweating. Fu Zi pattern: dark complexion, aversion to cold with cold limbs, pain and rigidity in lower back. Fu Zi pulse: sunken and faint) Based upon the patient's constitution pattern combined with the presence of the principal shàoyīn symptoms (faint, thin pulse and desire to sleep), I prescribed Ma Huang Fu Zi Gan Cao Tang plus Fu Zi Tang to warm yáng, dispel cold, disinhibit dampness, and remove impediments. I garnered two critical insights from this case:

Beginner students often think that diagnosis and treatment must strictly proceed according to the process of "identifying principles, devising methods, choosing a formula, and prescribing medicinals", but in reality, there is another diagnostic process that proceeds in precisely the opposite order (from medicinals, to formulas, to methods to principles). In this case, I based my diagnosis primarily on the patient's herb constitution pattern and formula pattern, combining these two diagnostic models in a synergistic approach.

Ma Huang Fu Zi Gan Cao Tang and Fu Zi Tang both treat shàoyīn impediment pain. In this case, I used both of these formulas. Ma Huang Fu Zi Gan Cao Tang warms yáng, resolves exterior contraction and lightly promotes sweating to treat yáng vacuity exterior contraction. Fu Zi Tang is known as a shàoyīn formula that consolidates the root and protects from exterior evil invasion. It treats, "shàoyīn disease with body pain, cold in the hands and feet and joint pain" and "lack of thirst with aversion to cold in the back". By combining Ma Huang Fu Zi Gan Cao tang and Fu Zi Tang, the ability to alleviate shàoyīn impediment pain is amplified. Ke Qin stated: "The Ma Huang Fu Zi Gan Cao Tang and Fu Zi Tang patterns are both shàoyīn exterior contraction patterns with heat effusion, sunken pulse, no interior (read: yīn conformation) symptoms and they develop as a result of cold penetrating from the yáng exterior into the channels. The body pain, joint pain, cold in hands and feet, aversion to cold on the back and sunken pulse are all the result of penetrating from the yīn interior into the bones. Ma Huang and Xi Xin target the cold penetrating from the yáng exterior into the channels, while Ren Shen, Fu Ling, Bai Zhu and Bai Shao target the penetration from the yīn interior into the bones. When there is no thirst and no heat in the trunk of the body, Fu Zi can always be used."

HIVD Treated with Wu Zhu Yu Tang
plus Dang Gui Si Ni Tang plus Fu Zi Tang
(Juéyīn-Shàoyīn Combination Disease Type)

MR. WANG, 32 YEARS

FIRST VISIT: January 21st, 2001

The patient fell from height and sustained a blunt force injury to his lower back three years ago. Recently, the pain in his lower back has increased and there is pain and numbness in his gluteal region and legs. He was diagnosed with HIVD and L4 spondylolysis via x-ray and CT scan.

CURRENT: The patient has a thin build and a drawn, pallid complexion. He relates that he has pain and coldness in his lower back with reduced mobility and dull pain radiating from his lumbosacral region down his leg. He has pain and numbness in his legs with reduced mobility that is worse in the left leg. He has increased lordosis in his lumbar spine and concavity in the lumbosacral region. His L4-S1 interspinous ligament is torn. Additionally, he complains of aversion to wind, profuse sweating, occasional dry heaving, frequent nausea, coldness, and discomfort in his stomach and distended pain in the crown of his head.

TONGUE: Engorged, scalloped pale and dark with a thick white coating.

PULSE: Thin and rough

ABDOMINAL PALPATION: The abdominal muscles are very thin and the rectus abdominis is rigid and contracted.

159

DIAGNOSIS: This is a juéyīn-shàoyīn combination disease impediment syndrome with counterflow of liver qì and rheum. There is simultaneous exterior cold congealing in the Juéyīn channel and interior cold damp congealing in shàoyīn at the lower back. Treatment should focus on warming yáng, supplementing qì, dispelling cold, eliminating dampness, warming the middle, and descending counterflow. This is precisely the function of Wu Zhu Yu Tang plus Dang Gui Si Ni Tang plus Fu Zi Tang: Wu Zhu Yu, Dang Shen, Gui Zhi, Dang Gui, Bai Shao, Fu Zi, Bai Zhu, Fu Ling all 10g, Xi Xin 5g, Tong Cao 5g, Gan Cao 5g, Da Zao 3 pieces, Sheng Jiang 5 slices. (Three packets)

I also performed bone-setting manipulations to rectify the lumbar vertebrae spinous process subluxations and used massage to address the torn interspinous ligament.

After treatment, the patient's lumbosacral pain intensified, he was unable to twist at the waist and was confined to his bed. After careful consideration of all aspects of the case, I concluded that I had not been mistaken in my diagnosis and prescription and prescribed another five packets of the same formula. I continued to massage the lumbosacral area and applied acupuncture and moxibustion at BL32, which had been particularly sensitive to pressing.

After treatment, the patient's lower back and leg pain steadily diminished, the distention and pain in the crown of the head, and cold in the stomach completely resolved, nausea and vomiting, and limb coldness decreased, but he still complained of bitterness in the mouth, dry throat, hot agitation, and aversion to wind.

ABDOMINAL PALPATION: The abdominal muscles were flat, rigid, and tight, there was propping binding at the chest and rib side, the sub-sternum felt tight and there were palpitations at the navel.

PULSE: sunken and wiry

TONGUE: thin, yellow coating.

DIAGNOSIS: The disease had already pivoted from yīn to yáng and become a shàoyáng-tàiyáng combination disease.

I prescribed Chai Hu Gui Zhi Tang and advised the patient to moxa the lower back, glutes and legs at points sensitive to pressure every day. After two months of treatment, the patient's lower back and leg pain gradually diminished. On a follow-up one year later, the patient reported that they made a complete recovery and were walking just like they had before the injury.

CLINICAL INSIGHT

Intermingling of yīn and yáng, co-dependent growth and decline of yīn and yáng, and counterflow and normalization of yīn and yáng are the three principal features of the Juéyīn conformation. After prescribing the patient Wu Zhu Yu Tang plus Dang Gui Si Ni Tang plus Fu Zi Tang based on a diagnosis of juéyīn-shàoyīn combination disease, the patient had a mìnxuàn reaction. However, I continued using the same formula, and after the second course of herbs, the patient's nausea resolved, crown of head pain diminished, and the disease pivoted from yīn to yáng. When the disease pivoted from Juéyīn and shàoyīn to tàiyáng and shàoyáng, the main symptom presentation was consistent with a Chai Hu Gui Zhi Tang formula pattern. After taking herbs for two months, the condition slowly resolved. I derived three insights from this case:

When treating HIVD, one must also be attentive to the dynamic progression of the disease, understand its general pattern of development but be cognizant of the possibility for variation, treat with herbal medicine and acumoxa, and craft treatments that mirror the movement of upright qì. Only in so doing can one truly put the unique features of six-conformation diagnosis into play.

The *Classic of History* (shàngshū, 尚書) states that "in intractable diseases, there can be no cure without a mìnxuàn reaction." In my humble opinion, mìnxuàn reactions represent a wavering of the stability of the diseased state and a sign of the return of upright qì.

A holistic view of the body should include a sense of how the whole exerts a guiding role on local processes as well as a sense of how local processes can influence the whole. Combining external and internal techniques is an important method of holistic therapy. Just as Xu Lingtai once stated: "If one does not grasp external therapy methods, then even if the disease is cured through herbs, one will only know one half of this medicine." (Impediment disease chapter of *Xu Ling-tai's Commentary on the Clinical Instruction and Case Studies*) (徐批臨證指南醫案·痹)

Osteoporosis Treated with Jin Gui Shen Qi Wan (Kidney Yáng Deficiency Type)

Ms. WANG, 55 YEARS

FIRST VISIT: September 15th, 1993

HISTORY: Ten years ago, the patient experienced periodic paralysis of the limbs due to hypokalemia and was successfully treated using western and Chinese medicine. Her blood tests all came back normal, but she developed chronic back pain. Through x-ray, she was found to have osteopenia in her thoracic and lumbar vertebrae as well as her pelvis and was diagnosed with osteoporosis.

CURRENT: The patient complains of feeling cold, having cold limbs, pain in the back, weakness of the knees, inability to stand or walk for extended periods of time, and even feeling discomfort after lying down for too long. Additionally, the patient reports feeling lazy and desiring sleep, but she claims to have a good appetite and normal BMs and urine. She entered post-menopause four years ago.

PULSE: Sunken and thin

TONGUE: Pale, tender, engorged, and scalloped.

PALPATION: Tenderness at bilateral sacroiliac joints, DU4 and the pubic symphysis.

In Chinese medical terminology, the patient's condition can be classified as bone impediment or bone wasting and is due to kidney yáng vacuity. The patient disliked the taste of decoctions, so I prescribed her Jin Gui Shen Qi Wan in pill form (twice daily, 12g each time). Additionally, I massaged areas that were sensitive to touch.

After five months of taking Shen Qi Wan, the patient's back pain completely resolved, and x-ray revealed that her bone density had noticeably improved. I advised her to continue taking the formula at a lower dose to reinforce the effects of treatment. On a follow-up five years later, she reported that she was able to complete house chores without discomfort.

CLINICAL INSIGHT

The kidney stores essence and presides over growth and development. In old age, kidney qì gradually diminishes, the kidney is unable to transform essence and becomes vacuous, leading to languishment of the bones and sinews. Epidemiological research in China has found that patients with kidney vacuity have lower levels of bone mineral content than healthy individuals and non-kidney vacuity patients. Given that the patient was also post-menopausal, her tiānguǐ water had dried and signs of kidney yáng vacuity were readily apparent, the first-choice formula was clearly an extended course of Shen Qi Wan to recover the body's original vitality. Interestingly, the patient had pain upon pressing at DU4, RN2 (pubic symphysis), and BL32 (sacroiliac joint). All these points are either directly or indirectly related to the kidney, which makes sense given the patient had kidney yáng and life gate fire vacuity. Massaging these points helps to speed up the absorption of the herbs and the rate of recovery.

Uterine Prolapse Treated with Dang Gui Si Ni Tang

35 YEARS, FEMALE

The patient developed frequent urination, urinary retention, and fullness and distention in the lower abdomen and was diagnosed by Western medicine with female urethral syndrome and stage 3 uterine prolapse, G3P1A2. She was advised to seek treatment with Chinese medicine. Previous doctors gave large doses of Bu Zhong Yi Qi Tang, Gui Pi Tang, Sheng Xian Tang etc., but her condition failed to improve. She was introduced to my clinic by a friend.

CURRENT: November 5th, 1999

The patient has a thin build and a sallow, dark complexion. She complains of palpitations, cold limbs, coldness, distention and pain in the lower back, headache, and aversion to wind. Her BMs are dry and hard at first and then sloppy and unformed. Urine is clear, frequent, scant, and there is some urinary retention. She feels discomfort in the lower abdomen upon standing that is relieved after lying down.

PULSE: Thin and weak

TONGUE: dark, pale red

ABDOMINAL PALPATION: The abdominal skin is quite thin and the rectus abdominis feels contracted on deep palpation.

Based upon the patient's coldness, distention and pain in the back, and BMs that started hard and ended sloppy, I first prescribed two weeks of Gui Zhi Tang plus Shen Zhuo Tang. Despite improving her palpitations, cold limbs, headache, aversion to cold, and back distention and pain, her lower abdomen discomfort, prolapse, urinary frequency, scantness, and retention got worse.

After careful consideration, I prescribed Gui Zhi Tang plus Wu Ling San, but this also proved to be off the mark. After a thorough analysis of the case, I was still unable to arrive at a satisfying diagnosis, so I went back to my books to consult the experience of my predecessors.

I found a case by Edo Period *kampo* master Masuo Utsugi's (宇津木 昆台) *Medical Transmission of Ancient Knowledge* (古訓醫傳) in which he treats a uterine prolapse patient with "coldness in the limbs and a thin and nearly expiring pulse" with Dang Gui Si Ni Tang. This case was very enlightening to me. Later on, I also realized that my diagnosis had been off the mark through my reading of Keisetsu Ōtsuka. I thus decided to prescribe Dang Gui Si Ni Tang:

Dang Gui 10g, Gui Zhi 10g, Bai Shao 10g, Xi Xin 3g, Gan Cao 3g, Tong Cao 5g, Da Zao 5 pieces. (Seven packets)

After finishing the herbs, the cold, distention, and pain effecting the patient's back as well as the lower abdominal discomfort improved and her BMs normalized, but the urinary frequency and scantness, cold hands and feet, and uterine prolapse were the same. I went with the same formula, adding Wu Zhu Yu 5g and Sheng Jiang 5 slices for another seven packets.

This formula was much more effective, and the patient decided to take another seven packets herself before returning to my clinic. She reported that the uterine prolapse was greatly improved and would only protrude with heavy labor. I prescribed another ten packets of Dang Gui Si Ni plus Wu Zhu Yu Sheng Jiang Tang.

After that last prescription I lost contact with the patient, but in the summer of the year 2000, a relative of hers to whom she had recommended my clinic informed me that she had made a complete recovery.

CLINICAL INSIGHT

For patients with multiple primary symptoms, eight-principle pattern differentiation is easy enough but selecting the right formula pattern requires careful thought and one can easily be lead astray. In such cases, it's extremely important to perform careful differential diagnosis of similar patterns and consult the clinical experience of our predecessors.

We are all quite familiar with Dang Gui Si Ni Tang and Dang Gui Si Ni plus Wu Zhu Yu, Sheng Jiang Tang and we know it's principally used to treat exterior contraction with cold hands and feet, but sometimes such thinking leads us to become too entrenched in one way of using the formula. The consequence of this is that we sometimes forget the formula and feel clueless when faced with the Dang Gui Si Ni Tang pattern in its protean clinical manifestations. So, in jīngfāng medicine, we must constantly update our knowledge, read widely, expand our horizons, and try to live up to the Confucian entreaty, "If you can improve yourself in a day, do so each day, forever building on prior improvements."

Infertility Subsequent to Induced Abortion Treated with Ge Gen Qin Lian Tang plus Gui Zhi Fu Ling Wan

MS. L, 35 YEARS (158CM, 55KG)

FIRST VISIT: October 2nd, 2014

CC: Infertility for 5 years

HISTORY: After multiple abortions, the patient developed infertility that failed to respond to multiple forms of Chinese and western medical therapy. A nationally famous gynecology specialist advised her to give up on treatment and find a surrogate mother because her endometrium was too thin (2mm) and it would be difficult to get pregnant even if she used IVF. When she heard this news, she broke down in tears. She said if she was unable to get pregnant it might cause a crisis in her marriage. The following year, she became a vegetarian, recited *The Original Vows of Ksitigarbha Bodhisattva Sutra* daily, released animals from captivity, performed good acts, and went to temples everywhere to pray to Buddha, but this also failed to reverse her infertility. Later on, she heard that many women who prayed to the Taoist Fertility Goddess Songzi Niangniang at Hua Mountain had been cured of infertility, so she made the pilgrimage to Shaanxi to offer her prayers there. With a devout heart, she embarked on her hike from the foot of Hua Shan, kowtowing three times with every step, all the way to the temple at Hua Shan's peak. In the process, she kowtowed so many times that she developed a massive blister on her forehead. At the summit, she met a woman who had gotten pregnant after praying to Songzi Niangniang and had returned to offer her thanks. She was also from Wenzhou and after suffering from infertility for many years, she had finally gotten pregnant after praying to Songzi Niangniang and taking my formulas. The woman recommended that the patient could visit me at my clinic when she returned from Shaanxi.

CURRENT: The patient has an average build and a dark red complexion. The blister from her trip to Shaanxi is still visible. She complains of bitterness of the mouth, halitosis, agitation and vexation, several BMs per day with sticky, sloppy stool, yellow, malodorous urine, tightness and rigidity in the neck, and acne throughout the back. She reports scant menses with dripping up to 10 days and yellow, profuse, malodorous leukorrhea.

TONGUE: Red with a yellow coating

PULSE: Slippery and rapid

ABDOMINAL PALPATION: strong springiness in the abdomen, substernal glomus, and pain upon pressing at the lower right and left quadrants.

DIAGNOSIS: Ge Gen Qin Lian Tang plus Gui Zhi Fu Ling Wan Pattern

FORMULA: First use Ge Gen Qin Lian Tang: Ge Gen 30g, Huang Lian 6g, Huang Qin 10g, Gan Cao 5g. (Fifteen packets, one per day, rest one day after taking five packets)

SECOND VISIT: October 21st

The patient reported that after taking the herbs, all symptoms had improved, especially the vexation and agitation.

FORMULA: Ge Gen Qin Lian Tang plus Gui Zhi Fu Ling Wan: Ge Gen 30g, Huang Lian 6g, Huang Qin 10g, Gan Cao 5g, Gui Zhi 10g, Fu Ling 20g,

Mu Dan Pi 10g, Chi Shao 15g, Tao Ren 1og. (Fifteen packets, one per day, rest one day after taking five packets)

THIRD VISIT: November 11th

I continued to use the same formula and prescribed fifteen packets, one per day with a rest day after every five packets as before. After two months of taking herbs, the patient successfully got pregnant. The patient was absolutely overjoyed and wrote a detailed summary that was several pages in length of the entire treatment process for me to express her gratitude.

Here is an excerpt of what she wrote:

"After taking your herbs, I noticed that I began having more flatulence, which I took to be a sign of detoxification. I also gained 2kg and my appetite improved—in the past I had suffered from coldness in my stomach. I really must thank you for advising me not to go for ultrasounds during the course of treatment. No doctor had ever done that before and I really felt a lot more relaxed! When my period didn't come in November, I didn't think much of it because my period is often irregular, and I hadn't taken any ovulation induction medicine. When I found out on December 12th that I was pregnant, aside from being filled with joy, I also found it all to be a bit unbelievable because my western doctor had told me that I had a low ovary reserve, a blocked left fallopian tube, and my endometrium was too thin. How could it be that all those problems had been resolved in such a short amount of time? An ultrasound conducted on January 3rd of 2015 revealed that the heart had developed in the embryo, which now measured 10mm and there were no abnormalities detected. I have the utmost gratitude for Ksitigarbha Bodhisattva, Dr. Lou and your daughter! I wish you all well!"

After delivering her child, the patient sent the following text message: "My son was born on July 29th, 2015, weighing 3.5kg. He has a thick head of black hair and fair, clear skin. Even though he didn't get washed on the first day after delivery, he still looks very clean and unwrinkled."

After eight months, she sent me another text message: "My son is now 8 months old and nearly 10kg. He's a very well-behaved little boy. Thank you so much Dr. Lou for your careful treatment. You made my dream of getting pregnant come true!"

CLINICAL INSIGHT

From this case, we can see the necessity of using jīngfāng style holistic diagnosis and treatment in infertility. If I had approached this case from the perspective of disease-based diagnosis and treatment, I might have thought to use Gui Zhi Fu Ling Wan, but I never would have considered using Ge Gen Qin Lian Tang. However, from the perspective of formula pattern diagnosis, it could not have been more obvious that Ge Gen Qin Lian Tang was the proper formula. As such, the comprehensive theory of disease and generalized treatment strategies developed in the *Treatise on Cold Damage* allow us to focus in on the specific presentations of formula patterns that we would otherwise ignore if we approached the patient from the perspective of disease-based diagnosis and treatment.

Below are the symptom presentations that led me to select Ge Gen Qin Lian Tang and Gui Zhi Fu Ling Wan:

Ge Gen Qin Lian Tang: Rigidity of the neck and upper back, bitter taste in the mouth, yellow urine, substernal glomus, palpitations, vexation, and diarrhea.

Gui Zhi Fu Ling Wan: Menstrual irregularity, dark red complexion, springiness in the abdomen, pain upon pressing in lower left quadrant.

There is nothing wrong with specialization in Chinese hospitals per se, but Chinese doctors shouldn't carry this idea of specialization into their diagnosis. The wisdom of the *Treatise on Cold Damage*'s "formula pattern correspondence" and "treating according to pattern" should be a basic skill taught to all Chinese doctors. For the majority of Chinese doctors that already have a strong grasp of disease-targeted diagnosis and treatment, studying the generalized treatment strategy of the *Treatise on Cold Damage* is absolutely imperative. As Taiwanese cultural critic Sun Ji-long (孫隆基) put it in *The Deep Structure of Chinese Culture* (中國文化的深層結構), "Gaining another perspective from which to view things brings us one step closer to the truth. It might be impossible to know for sure if something is the truth, but it can be intuited as such."

The above is just a summary of one infertility case, but in clinic, it is our standard practice to treat all infertility cases using formula pattern diagnosis. Over several decades of practice, I've successfully treated over 100 cases of infertility. In the past two years alone, we've treated over ten cases successfully. In 1995, I wrote a summary of my experience using formula pattern diagnosis in this disease which was titled *Clinical Case Studies Using Jīngfāng formulas to Treat Fertility Based on Abdominal Diagnosis*. That was also the year that Beijing hosted the fourth annual World Conference on Women. During that time, I presented seven cases using formula pattern diagnosis to treat infertility at the National Chinese Medicine Gynecology Symposium in the NGO CSW conference. Transcripts from that symposium were later made publicly available.

This infertility case features the successful use of a non-disease-specific treatment strategy. This demonstrates that formula pattern correspondence is a viable alternative to disease-targeted or mechanism-based diagnosis and treatment strategies. This cases also reminds us of an important, if commonly understood fact: As far as Chinese medicine is concerned, diseases do not follow any predictable model. Philosophers have often said something similar: Nature has no plan, and history never plays out according to script.

Infertility with Advanced Menstruation Treated with Gui Zhi Tang (Tàiyáng Type)

Ms. Zhang, 26 years

FIRST VISIT: October 7th, 1985

HISTORY: The patient has been infertile for three years. She had her first period at 16-years-old and has always had advanced menstruation, copious volume, long duration and light-colored thin menses. Biphasic basal body temperature is intact, the follicular stage is relatively short, and she has corpus luteum insufficiency.

CURRENT: The patient has a thin build, looks fatigued, and has a pallid facial complexion. She complains of longstanding aversion to cold, spontaneous sweating, and slight heat effusion. Her body temperature is normal.

PULSE: Floating, soggy, and slightly rapid

TONGUE: Pale red with a thin, greasy coating

ABDOMINAL PALPATION: No remarkable findings

I diagnosed this as tàiyáng disease wind-strike syndrome and prescribed three packets of Gui Zhi Tang to resolve the flesh, expel wind, harmonize construction and defense, and warm and contain menstrual blood.

Gui Zhi 10g, Bai Shao 10g, Zhi Gan Cao 10g, Da Zao 5 pieces, Sheng Jiang 5 slices. Needle GB20 (Bilateral), BL12 (Bilateral)

After the herbs and acupuncture, the patient's aversion to cold slightly diminished, spontaneous sweating was partially reigned in, spontaneous sweating was less noticeable, and the pulse was floating, soggy but not rapid. I added Dang Gui 10g, Chuan Xiong 6g and prescribed another seven packets. That month, her period came on time with a normal volume and a dark red color. She still felt some aversion to wind and spontaneous sweating. I used the same formula for another two weeks with the doses of Gui Zhi and Bai Shao halved. After two weeks, all symptoms resolved, and I had her suspend treatment and monitor her condition. The next month she had a successful conception and later gave birth to her first child.

CLINICAL INSIGHT

Apart from having unique patterns of development and etiologies, diseases also have shared, generalized etiologies—fertility is no different. Using febrile disease as a point of entry, the *Treatise on Cold Damage* is an analysis of common patterns of pathological responses of the body to disease and a record of non-disease targeted methodologies to treat these pathological manifestations. This is why later commentators would go on to say, "No disease is outside the purview of the six-conformation system" and "The theory propounded in the *Treatise on Cold Damage* can be applied to all diseases". In his preface to the *Treatise*, Zhong-jing said of the generalized pattern of diagnosis and treatment he developed: "Though it might not be able to cure all diseases, it will at least allow you to understand the source of the diseases you encounter...Those who apply my method in clinic are knowledgeable and insightful." By the Jin and Yuan dynasties, over a millennium after the publishing of the *Treatise*, physicians began to understand the book as a "general theory of all disease". What they meant by a "general theory of all disease" was a theory that delineated a generalized system of diagnosis and treatment based upon observable patterns. Chinese medicine, which places great import on the "unity of heaven and mankind" and "harmony and holism", puts more emphasis on its generalized system of common patterns of disease than modern medicine. When the *Inner Cannon* speaks of "being versed in principle and logic" it is asking that physicians integrate medical principles (diagnosis and treatment based on the generalized system of common patterns of pathological manifestation) and medical logic (diagnosis and treatment based upon unique features of individual diseases). When comparing medical principle and medical logic, we must be aware that "the logic of all things is encompassed in the great principles." (Han Feizi) That is, it is without question that medical principle assumes the guiding role in Chinese medical practice.

From a six-conformation diagnosis perspective, this patient had longstanding tàiyáng wind strike syndrome. Despite having "aversion to wind, spontaneous sweating, and slight heat effusion", her temperature was normal, so other physicians didn't pick up on it. Because I had a clear grasp of the longstanding tàiyáng wind strike syndrome symptom presentation and also placed importance on the patient's herb constitution pattern (thin build, pallid complexion, aversion to wind, and spontaneous sweating are all indicative of a Gui Zhi constitution), after considering these various factors, I chose to prescribe Gui Zhi Tang. By combining Chinese herbs and acupuncture, and correctly matching the presentation to the Gui Zhi Tang formula pattern, I was able to quickly rectify her longstanding advanced menstruation condition. Once her menstrual cycle was rectified, she was able to successfully conceive soon after.

Infertility with Menstrual Diarrhea Treated with Gan Cao Xie Xin Tang (Shàoyáng Type)

Ms. Li, 32 years

FIRST VISIT: May 7th, 1985

The patient has had infertility for five years. Following an abortion in September of 1980, the patient began having delayed menstruation with average volume, light-colored, thin menses that lasted for one week. She has a typical biphasic basal body temperature with stepwise midcycle temperature rise. Her cycle typically lasts 60 days with a 44–45 day follicular phase and an 8–9 day luteal phase. During her period, she has borborygmus and diarrhea which resolves at the end of the period.

CURRENT: The patient also complains of stomach distention, glomus and fullness, stomach clamoring and eructation, sloppy and unformed stools, poor sleep quality, agitation, and frequent canker sores.

PULSE: Wiry

TONGUE: Pale red with a thin, yellow, and greasy coating

ABDOMINAL PALPATION: Substernal hard glomus, pain upon pressing at DU9, but continued massage at the point produces comfort in the sub-sternum.

DIAGNOSIS: Stomach cold with intestinal heat. This is a mixed replete-vacuity shàoyáng glomus syndrome.

FORMULA: Gan Cao Xie Xin Tang: Zhi Gan Cao 10g, Ban Xia 10g, Huang Qin 5g, Gan Jiang 5g, Huang Lian 3g, Da Zao 5 pieces, Dang Shen 10g. (Fifteen packets)

Additionally, I advised her to have a family member massage DU9 twelve times per day for 30s.

SECOND VISIT: Substernal glomus was reduced, frequency of menstrual diarrhea was noticeably diminished, there was a slight abatement of pain upon pressing at DU9, and stools were still slightly unformed.

I continued using this formula with a slightly reduced dose until July, after which I told the patient she could suspend treatment and monitor her condition. At the end of September the same year, she was found to be pregnant during a gynecological exam and gave birth to a healthy baby girl in May of the next year.

CLINICAL INSIGHT

Six-conformation diagnosis is a patient-focused clinical system guided by yīn-yáng theory. Yīn-yáng theory is used to elucidate changes to the pathological state of the whole body in varying stages of disease as opposed to focusing on specific etiologies or sites of disease. This approach focuses on the current pathological picture in a dynamic and unfolding process of disease as opposed to the static, underlying causative factors.

For instance, in this case, previous physicians failed because they only focused on the local sites of dysfunction in the viscera-bowels and channels. They only looked for etiologies in the thoroughfare vessel, controlling vessel, liver, and kidneys and neglected to seek an understanding of the wholistic nature of the disease in terms of the six conformations.

"Substernal hard glomus" is the primary symptom for Xie Xin Tang family formulas, but this finding must be considered alongside other key symptoms like poor sleep quality and agitation to narrow the pattern down to Gan Cao Xie Xin Tang. Clearly, abdominal diagnosis is not in conflict with the four examinations.

Infertility with Primary Dysmenorrhea Treated with Tao He Cheng Qi Tang plus Da Huang Fu Zi Tang (Tàiyáng-Yángmíng Combination Disease Type)

Ms. Wang, 30 years

FIRST VISIT: July 21st, 1982

HISTORY: Ever since the patient's menarche at 15, she has experienced a stabbing pain radiating from her lower left abdomen to below her left rib and down her left lower back and leg respectively during her period. Her period is regular with a low volume, uneven flow, and dark, purple, clotted menses. After getting married, all symptoms worsened, and she has been unable to conceive in seven years of marriage. She was diagnosed with primary dysmenorrhea and infertility by Western medicine. Chinese medical physicians previously prescribed Shao Fu Zhu Yu Tang and other blood stasis dispelling formulas with poor results.

CURRENT: Despite having a full, robust figure, the patient's complexion is dark and pallid. She complains of constipation.

PULSE: Wiry and rough

TONGUE: Pale, purple, and scalloped with a thick, white, watery coating.

ABDOMINAL PALPATION: The abdomen is robust and full, the rectus abdominis is tight and contracted on both sides, there is a tight bind in the lower left abdomen that is painful to the touch and the left rib side is full and uncomfortable.

DIAGNOSIS: This is a replete congealed cold and blood stasis pattern

FORMULA: Tao He Cheng Qi Tang plus Da Huang Fu Zi Tang: Tao Ren 10g, Gui Zhi 15g, Da Huang 6g, Gan Cao 6g, Yuan Ming Fen 10g (dissolve), Fu Zi 10g, Xi Xin 5g (add to decoction at end) (Seven packets)

Additionally, I advised her to moxa the bind in her lower left abdomen twice a day for 15 minutes each time.

After completing the course of herbs and moxa, her BMs normalized to once per day, the bind in her left lower abdomen disappeared, but was still painful upon deep pressure. Additionally, she still had some contraction and tightness in the rectus abdominis. Given this presentation, I pivoted to a Gui Zhi Fu Ling Wan modification. After taking thirty-five packets and using moxa every day, all symptoms resolved, her menstrual pain vanished, and I advised her to suspend treatment and monitor her condition. In October of 1982 she successfully conceived and had a smooth delivery the following year.

CLINICAL INSIGHT

The patient had a clear blood stasis presentation, but previous attempts to use blood- quickening formulas had been unsuccessful. There are several reasons why this could have happened, but I think a key reason is that they ignored the patient's abdominal presentation. The lower left abdomen pain that radiated to the lower back and left leg corresponds to the Da Huang Fu Zi Tang abdominal pattern characterized by radiating "pain on one side below the ribs" in the *Essential Prescriptions*, and the Tao He Cheng Qi Tang abdominal pattern characterized by "urgent binding in the lower left or right abdomen that is averse to touch" in the *Treatise on Cold Damage*. The Japanese *kampo* physician Takahide Kuwaki (桑木崇秀) stated that all lower abdominal (especially lower left) pain upon pressing and palpable binds could be treated with Gui Zhi Fu Ling Wan. Otsuka Keisetsu, Dōmei Yakazu, Takahide Kuwaki, and other twentieth century *kampo* practitioners all seemed to espouse this view. The fact that I was able to achieve success in this case based upon abdominal diagnosis alone gives credence to Yoshimasu Tōdō (吉益東洞), who once said: "If the abdominal presentation is not conclusive, a formula should not be prescribed."

Infertility with Premenstrual Anxiety Treated with Zhu Ling Tang (Yángmíng Type)

MS. LIU, 27 YEARS

FIRST VISIT: September 15th, 1983

The patient has a thin build. In four years of marriage, she has yet to conceive. Her menses are dark red, normal volume, and absent of clots. Around ten days before her period, she begins to develop agitation, vexation, headache, vertigo, nausea or vomiting, breast tenderness, diarrhea, and lower limb edema. These symptoms all abate with the beginning of her period.

When she arrived at my clinic, she happened to be right at the peak of premenstrual symptoms. She additionally complained of dry mouth, a slight cough, and yellow, inhibited urine.

PULSE: Wiry, thin, and rapid

TONGUE: Red with a thin yellow coating

ABDOMINAL PALPATION: The entire lower abdomen is distended and full and there are palpitations below the navel.

DIAGNOSIS: This is water and heat blocking the bāo (胞)[14] with vacuity of yīn and fluid.

---

[14] Can refer to either the uterus or the bladder. Here it would seem that both are appropriate.

FORMULA: Zhu Ling Tang: Zhu Ling 15g, Fu Ling 15g, Ze Xie 15g, E Jiao 10g (dissolve), Hua Shi 12g. (Seven packets)

Additionally, I advised the patient to moxa RN6 and RN4 for ten minutes twice daily.

After the above course of herbs and moxa, all symptoms gradually diminished. I advised her to take Zhu Ling Tang for seven days starting ten days before her period and moxa RN4 and RN3. After three months of treatment, the patient's condition completely resolved. In May of the following year, the patient conceived and later gave birth to healthy baby boy.

CLINICAL INSIGHT

There are several possible causes of premenstrual anxiety, but they are more or less rooted in a similar mechanism relating to premenstrual physiology. In the days leading up to a woman's period, peaking progesterone levels cause an increase in sodium and water retention leading to an electrolyte imbalance, and a subsequent increase in extracellular fluid and edema. The edema not only occurs on the surface of the body, but also around the internal organs, including the brain, which is what accounts for the premenstrual headaches and anxiety.

From a six-channel perspective, this patient had a yángmíng heat-water bind Zhu Ling Tang pattern. Yángmíng is characterized by "dry metal". The Book of Changes (易經) states, "Fire is attracted to dryness", while Explaining the Hexagrams (說卦) states, "Of all things, nothing dries more than fire". Practical experience demonstrates that things close to a source of fire will be dry, while those further away will become damper. Therefore, yángmíng dry heat can be the primary cause of both fluid insufficiency and fluid accumulation. The patient's lower abdominal fullness and distention and sub-umbilical palpitations were both signs of a water congestion abdominal pattern. The stagnant water led to inhibited urine, the uneven distribution of water to the large intestine caused diarrhea, and water qì invading the stomach and lung led to vomiting and cough. Additionally, the inability of clear yáng to upbear caused headache and vertigo, while the inhibited qì flow led to impediment of the collaterals causing premenstrual breast edema and pain. Finally, yīn vacuity and the effulgent fire that scorched fluid, congealing it into phlegm, accounted for the patient's thin build, insomnia, vexation, red tongue, and rapid pulse. After considering the patient's abdominal presentation, pulse, tongue and symptomatic findings, I prescribed Zhu Ling Tang to nourish yīn and disinhibit water.

Infertility with Delayed Menstruation
Treated with Chai Hu Gui Zhi Gan Jiang Tang plus Dang Gui Shao Yao San (Shàoyáng-Tàiyīn Type)

Ms. Li, 27 years

FIRST VISIT: May 10th, 1984

After four years of marriage, the patient still hasn't successfully conceived. She reports having delayed menstruation with a 40–50 day cycle. She has scant menses and uneven flow. She also complains of breast distention and pain that starts one week prior to her period. She was diagnosed with PCOS and infertility by Western medicine.

CURRENT: The patient appears despondent and complains of palpitations, vexation, dry and bitter mouth with no desire to drink water, frequent sighing, tension and heaviness in the traps, poor appetite, sloppy stools and scant, yellow urine.

PULSE: Long, wiry, slippery

TONGUE: Pale red with a thick, greasy white coating

ABDOMINAL PALPATION: Discomfort and fullness in the chest and rib-side, palpitations above the navel, and pain throughout the periumbilical and lower left abdominal area upon pressing.

CHANNEL PALPATION: Pain upon pressing at DU2

DIAGNOSIS: Liver stagnation, rheum amassment, and blood stasis blocking the thoroughfare and controlling vessels.

FORMULA: Chai Hu Gui Zhi Gan Jiang Tang plus Dang Gui Shao Yao San: Chai Hu, Huang Qin, Dang Gui, Chi Shao, Chuan Xiong, Bai Zhu, Ze Xie all 10g, Gui Zhi 12g, Gan Jiang 5g, Sheng Mu Li 30g, Tian Hua Fen 12g, Fu Ling 15g.

Additionally, I wet cupped at DU2 and reassured the patient that her condition would improve to instill her with confidence in the treatment and help lighten her mood.

After thirty days of taking this formula and wet cupping three times at DU2, her symptoms steadily improved and premenstrual breast tenderness diminished. After taking the same formula for another two months, she finally successfully conceived in September of 1984 and gave birth to a baby boy the next year.

CLINICAL INSIGHT

Based upon the patient's bitter mouth, dry throat, vertigo, fullness and discomfort in the chest and rib-side, and wiry pulse, I diagnosed the patient with a shàoyáng disease Chai Hu pattern. Based on her reduced appetite, sloppy stools, frequent and scant urine, slight edema in the lower left leg, pale, red, and scalloped tongue with a white, greasy coating, and wiry, tight and slippery pulse, I concluded she simultaneously also had tàiyīn replete cold damp. As such, I prescribed her Chai Hu Gui Zhi Gan Jiang Tang to course and harmonize shàoyáng and warmly dispel tàiyīn cold. Because the patient also had delayed menstruation with scant volume indicating blood vacuity and an abdominal presentation resembling a Dang Gui Shao Yao San abdominal pattern, I prescribed her Dang Gui Shao Yao San to nourish and quicken blood and disinhibit water. Chai Hu Gui Zhi Gan Jiang Tang in combination with Dang

Gui Shao Yao San not only courses the channels and quickens blood to urgently treat the branch condition, it also nourishes blood and moves water to treat the root, thereby resolving the contradiction posed by the fact that blood vacuity leads to relatively replete water and dampness.

The Essential Prescriptions describes the abdominal pattern for Dang Gui Shao Yao San rather vaguely, offering only "gripping pain in the abdomen". In his *Extraordinary Views of Abdominal Patterns* (腹證奇覽), Inaba Katsu Bunrei (稻葉克文禮), shares his own understanding of the Dang Gui Shi Yao San abdominal pattern based on his extensive clinical experience: "Periumbilical contraction and pain upon pressing that radiates to the back". Bloodletting to unblock the collaterals was another important aspect of treatment in this case. This was a classic case of using external and internal treatment methods to achieve success.

Infertility with Excessive Leukorrhea Treated with High-Dose Zhen Wu Tang (Shàoyīn Type)

MS. SUN, 27 YEARS

FIRST VISIT: March 7th, 1985

HISTORY: The patient has failed to conceive after five years of marriage. She has consistently had copious, transparent leukorrhea and has been diagnosed by Western medicine with cervicitis, underdeveloped uterus, and ovarian insufficiency. She has a monophasic basal body temperature.

CURRENT: The patient appears fatigued and has dark circles under the eyes. She complains of frequent muscle spasm, palpitations, shortness of breath, sloppy and unformed stools, heaviness in the lower limbs with premenstrual pitting edema, slightly delayed menstruation, and scant, light-colored and thin menses.

PULSE: Soggy and thin

TONGUE: Pale, scalloped with a thick white coating.

ABDOMINAL PALPATION: The abdomen appears full and distended and is soft upon pressing with weak springiness. There are strong palpitations above the navel.

DIAGNOSIS: Shàoyīn yáng vacuity with water overspilling.

FORMULA: Zhen Wu Tang: Fu Zi 30g (decoct before other herbs for 30 minutes), Bai Shao 12g, Fu Ling 30g, Bai Zhu 15g, Sheng Jiang 5 slices. (10 packets)

Additionally, I advised the patient to moxa at RN9 (where palpitations were palpable) for 15 minutes per day.

After this course of herbs and moxa, the patient's leukorrhea diminished and all other symptoms also improved. I prescribed the same formula again over the course of several weeks for a total of 50 packets. In the beginning of June, the patient developed a biphasic basal body temperature and by the end of July, she had successfully conceived. Because the patient had slight pain upon pressure in her lower left abdomen and occasionally had lower leg edema, I prescribed her Dang Gui Shao Yao San to be taken intermittently for two months. In March of 1986, she successfully gave birth to a baby boy.

CLINICAL INSIGHT

The patient's symptoms, including her copious and transparent leukorrhea, cold limbs, palpitations, and sloppy stools, were all consistent with a shàoyīn true fire vacuity and kidney yáng vacuity with overspilling water qì pathology. Based upon famous Chinese medical gynecologist Zhao Song-quan's (趙松泉) theory "the first half of the menstrual cycle is related to yīn, while the latter half of the menstrual cycle is related to yáng", I diagnosed her monophasic basal temperature as an indication of yáng qì vacuity. Based upon these findings, I prescribed Zhen Wu Tang with higher doses of Bai Zhu and Fu Zi and moxa on RN9 to powerfully supplement yáng and transform yīn cold. In my experience, abdominal findings can serve not only as a basis for diagnosis but can also be viewed as important targets for acupuncture and moxa.

In *Explanations of Kampo Formula Patterns* (漢方處方解證) *kampo* physician Dōmei Yakazu states: "*Kampo* medicine is distinguished by its focus on treating based on pattern. As such it can be called 'symptom and pattern medicine', 'formula pattern correspondence medicine' or even 'formula medicine'. The diagnosis of symptomatology is linked directly to the formula. The diagnosis is the treatment and thus the pattern is the formula." While treating this patient, I noted how closely their symptoms conformed to the descriptions of Zhen Wu Tang in the *Treatise on Cold Damage*: "Substernal palpitations, vertigo and spasms" and "when there is abdominal pain, inhibited urine, heaviness and pain in the limbs, and diarrhea, this is due to water qì...Zhen Wu Tang is indicated." These lines reflect the relationship between formula pattern diagnosis and symptomology, pathology, pharmacology, and therapeutics. This is why prescribing based upon formula patterns is effective.

Infertility with Amenorrhea Treated with Wen Jing Tang (Juéyīn Type)

Ms. Zhang, 32 years

FIRST VISIT: February 10th, 1984

HISTORY: The patient has failed to conceive in five years of marriage. Her menarche came at 18 years old and has subsequently had delayed menstruation, with periods only coming every three-four months. In the past eight months, she has developed amenorrhea, which Western medicine diagnosed as secondary amenorrhea (though the primary cause remained unclear). She was found to have a monophasic basal temperature.

CURRENT: The patient has a pale, dark complexion and complains of pain and cold in the lower abdomen, aversion to cold, cold limbs, dry lips, dry cracked palms, cold hands and feet, sloppy stools, and copious, transparent leukorrhea.

PULSE: Sunken and tight

TONGUE: Dark and pale with a thick, white, greasy coating.

ABDOMINAL PALPATION: Fullness and distention in the lower abdomen that is soft and lacks springiness. No binds can be palpated.

CHANNEL PALPATION: Pain upon pressing DU2.

DIAGNOSIS: Juéyīn disease, liver channel qì and blood stagnation, and yáng qì vacuity diffusion.

FORMULA: Wen Jing Tang: Dang Gui 10g, Ban Xia 10g, Mai Dong 1og, Dang Shen 15g, E Jiao 10g (Dissolved), Mu Dan Pi 6g, Chuan Xiong 6g, Gui Zhi 6g, Gan Cao 2g, Wu Zhu Yu 1.5g, Gan Jiang 3g.

Additionally, I wet cupped at DU2 every second week.

After fifty days of treatment, she developed a biphasic basal body temperature and showed signs of ovulation. She continued taking this formula and getting wet cupping, and ultimately conceived successfully in June of 1984.

CLINICAL INSIGHT

Intermingling of yīn and yáng, co-dependent growth and decline of yīn and yáng, and counterflow and normalization of yīn and yáng are the three principal characteristics of Juéyīn disease. Additionally, Juéyīn disease also often involves dysfunction of the coursing of liver qì and related blood disorders. The fact that the major Juéyīn formulas Dang Gui Si Ni Tang and Dang Gui Si Ni plus Wu Zhu Yu, Sheng Jiang Tang both feature Dang Gui in their names demonstrates the role of blood disorders in Juéyīn.

Wen Jing Tang can be seen as a modification of Dang Gui Si Ni Tang plus Wu Zhu Yu, Sheng Jiang. The formula appears in the "Miscellaneous Gynecological Diseases" chapter of the *Essential Prescriptions of the Golden Chamber* where it is indicated for "Urgency in the lower abdomen, abdominal fullness, heat vexation in the palms, dry lips and dry mouth... it also is indicated for coldness in the lower abdomen with infertility or advanced menstruation". Zhong-jing's classic blood nourishing and channel warming formula is marked by an abdominal presentation featuring coldness in the lower abdomen, lower abdominal distention and fullness, lack of springiness, and lack of binds or masses. The patient's presentation matched the formula pattern, so naturally it was effective in treating her infertility.

In amenorrhea, one can often find sensitive spots in the lumbosacral region and especially at DU2, DU3, and below the 5ᵗʰ lumbar vertebrae at EX-B8 (what the Japanese call "The High Immortal Point"). Wet cupping at these points will greatly improve the efficaciousness of treatment.

Menstruation is closely linked with the liver's blood-storing and coursing functions. It is Juéyīn that chiefly presides over this dynamic of storing and coursing, inbearing and outbearing. If vacuity cold is generated within and ice lodges in the sea of blood, infertility, and transparent cold leukorrhea often result. Thus, the Jin Dynasty physician Liu Wan-su (劉完素) stated: "The flow of tiānguǐ water should be understood in terms of Juéyīn function."

Infertility with Oligomenorrhea Treated with Shen Qì Wan (Kidney Qì Deficiency and Cold Congealing in the Thoroughfare and Conception Vessels Type)

MS. ZHANG, 26 YEARS

FIRST VISIT: October 5th, 1978

HISTORY: The patient has a history of infertility for three years with oligomenorrhea, scant, light-colored menses, and monophasic basal body temperature. Apart from a slightly narrow cervix, Western medicine examination did not reveal any remarkable findings. She was diagnosed with primary infertility and oligomenorrhea.

CURRENT: The patient appears fatigued and has a pallid complexion. She complains of soreness and pain in her knees.

TONGUE: Pale with a watery, white coating.

ABDOMINAL PALPATION: Her lower abdomen is soft and lacks springiness, and there is contraction along the conception vessel below the navel. A chopstick-thick bind can be felt below the navel.

DIAGNOSIS: This is kidney yáng vacuity with cold congealing in the conception and thoroughfare vessels.

TREATMENT: Shen Qì Wan in pill form, 10g taken twice daily.

Additionally, I advised her to moxa on RN4 and RN6 twice daily for 10–15 minutes.

After two weeks of moxa and herbs, symptoms began to improve and the contraction below the navel diminished. I continued to treat the patient in this way for another five months. During this time, her period slowly stabilized at 35 days, after which she developed a biphasic basal body temperature. On August 15ᵗʰ of 1979, she was found to be pregnant and gave birth in March of the next year to a baby girl.

CLINICAL INSIGHT

Infertility is a complex and multi-faceted disease with countless mechanisms, treatments, and formulas. I often approach infertility from a holistic perspective and place particular importance on the abdominal presentation. For instance, this patient's lower abdomen lacked springiness, she had contraction below the navel along the conception vessel, and chopstick-wide bind — these are the main characteristics of the Shen Qi Wan abdominal pattern. We were able to achieve a good result in this case by basing our herbal and moxa treatment on this abdominal formula pattern. However, in treating infertility, the physician must be patient and should not switch out a formula after a few packets if the effects are not immediately apparent.

Perimenopausal Symptoms Treated with Shen Qi Wan plus Zhi Bo Di Huang Wan (Kidney Essence and Yáng Vacuity)

Ms. LI, 50 YEARS

FIRST VISIT: March 5th, 1999

HISTORY: The patient has a history of vertigo for over one year and was diagnosed with perimenopausal disorder by Western medicine.

CURRENT: The patient has an average build and appears fatigued. She complains of cold limbs, desire for warmth, pain in the lower back, and frequent urination, but also sweats spontaneously, has poor sleep quality, and vivid dreams that connect over several days (she laughingly described this as her nightly soap opera viewing session). Her blood pressure trends low, and her periods come every 2–3 months with increasingly scant volume.

PULSE: Sunken and forceless

TONGUE: Pale red with a white, watery coating

ABDOMINAL PALPATION: The lower abdomen is soft, lacks springiness, and she says it sometimes feels numb.

DIAGNOSIS: Kidney essence and yáng vacuity, undernourishment of the conception and thoroughfare vessels, and empty vacuity of the brain marrow.

FORMULA: Shen Qi Wan plus Zhi Bo Di Huang Wan, 10g per day.

After a month of herbs, all symptoms improved, and her dreams were less vivid and frequent. After another two months using the same formula, her condition completely resolved. On a follow-up three years later, she said that on the odd occasion she felt a flare coming, she was able to manage it easily with the above formula.

CLINICAL INSIGHT

Western medicine asserts that perimenopausal disorder is primarily a kind of dysautonomia caused by overactivity of the pituitary gland and atrophy of the ovaries. There are western medical treatments available, but they are not always helpful and come with certain side effects. Chinese medicine believes that this disease is often due to kidney qì vacuity and the exhaustion of blood and yīn. It's often easy enough to diagnose, but it can require a long course of treatment and patients often tire of decocting herbs. As such, using the pill form of these formulas can increase patient compliance.

Using Shen Qi Wan plus Zhi Bo Di Huang Wan to treat the patient's vertigo corresponds to the *Simple Questions* notion of treating below when there is counterflow and the disease manifests above. (SW70) However, in my clinical practice these theoretical considerations are always secondary to formula pattern diagnostics. This patient's complaint of "numbness below the navel" corresponded to the description of the abdominal pattern for Shen Qi Wan described in the *Essential Prescriptions* as "numbness in the lower abdomen".

Pediatric Encephalitis Treated with Ge Gen Jia Ban Xia Tang

Ms. Chen, 3 years

The patient has had a consistent high fever for four days and a symptomatology marked by drowsiness, clouded spirit, and stiffness in the neck. A western medical hospital suspected she may have encephalitis, but the family would not allow a lumbar puncture to confirm diagnosis. She was treated for symptoms with western and Chinese medicine, but her condition continued to worsen, so her family brought her to my clinic for treatment.

CURRENT: The patient was drowsy and had a fever of 41°C. Her forehead was extremely hot to the touch, her feet were cold, and she had occasional explosive vomiting. Her pulse was rapid and floating. Her parents tried using cold compresses and fanning to drop her fever, but the patient had goosebumps, no sweating, and was averse to the wind and cold. Her tongue had a white, watery coating and her neck was rigid with a positive Kernig's sign.

Based upon her rigid neck, heat effusion, aversion to cold, no sweating, floating and rapid pulse, white and watery tongue coating, and vomiting, I gave Ge Gen Tang plus Ban Xia to resolve the flesh, promote sweating, upbear fluid, unblock the collaterals, check retching, and downbear counterflow.

FORMULA: Ge Gen 9g, Ma Huang 4.5g, Gui Zhi 3g, Bai Shao 6g, Sheng Gan Cao 3g, Da Zao 3 pieces, Sheng Jiang 6g.

I also told her parents that the high fever was just the body's attempt to eliminate the pathogen and there was no need to use external means to drop the fever.

Two hours after taking the herbs, the patient began sweating, her temperature dropped to 38°C, the vomiting abated, and she felt thirsty. I fanned her with a large fan and she no longer showed signs of aversion to wind and cold, but she was extremely fatigued, didn't want to be covered with a blanket, had yellow urine, was constipated, and her pulse became surging and large. I concluded that her condition had already shifted into yángmíng and, as the Qing dynasty physician Lu Maoxiu (陸懋修) noted, there are no lethal disorders in yángmíng, so the most dangerous stage of her illness had passed. I then gave two packets of Bai Hu Jia Ren Shen Tang, after which she made a complete recovery and experienced no lingering symptoms. In the above case, the patient didn't have access to IV fluids. If she did have access, she should have been put on an IV drip to maintain electrolyte balance.

Pediatric Exterior Contraction with Heat Effusion Treated with Ge Gen Tang plus Hua Shi

On a rainy day in the summer of 1982, my then 3-year-old daughter developed exterior contraction and heat effusion with a temperature of 38.5°C. She had a Ge Gen Tang presentation. That night at 6pm, I gave her a dose of Ge Gen Tang, after which she soon fell asleep. Around midnight, she suddenly woke up and started crying. Her face was flushed, she was agitated, not sweating, had a temperature of 39.5°C, was extremely thirsty, and drank several cups of water. I concluded that her condition had pivoted to a tàiyáng-yángmíng combination disease. Unfortunately, I didn't have any Shi Gao at home and no pharmacies would be open so late at night, so I had no choice but to use some talcum powder (Hua Shi) that I had on hand. After taking the decoction she once again fell asleep right away. I stayed by her side so that I could continually monitor her situation. Only after she developed a slight sweat, and her fever abated at three in the morning did I dare sleep. When I woke up the next morning at 8am, she was back to normal and bouncing around with energy. Soon after, my wife came into the bedroom and let out a shrill scream. My daughter's pillow was covered in blood. This, I reasoned, was the "red sweat" of my daughter's nosebleed.

Infant Episodic Colic Treated
with Gui Zhi Jia Gui Tang

5 MONTHS, MALE

FIRST VISIT: July 3rd, 2013

HISTORY: The patient was smoothly delivered, but two weeks ago began crying incessantly for no apparent reason. He would have multiple episodes of crying throughout each day and would awake from sleep to cry as well. Between episodes, the parents couldn't find anything wrong with the child. He was diagnosed by Western medicine with intermittent, episodic enterospasms. His parents tried to treat him using Tu Si Zi Teng (菟絲子籐), a popular remedy for colic in the southern Zhejiang region, but his condition persisted.

CURRENT: During episodes, the child's face becomes flushed, the abdomen gets distended and tight, and he rolls around in the fetal position, screeching in pain. When the abdomen becomes distended and full, one can see a protruding induration tracing the path of the colic pain on his stomach. When the protruding induration rolls to RN12, it suddenly disappears and the child stops crying.

ABDOMINAL PALPATION: The abdomen feels distended and full, with palpitations at the navel.

DIAGNOSIS: Running Piglet, Gui Zhi Jia Gui Tang pattern.

FORMULA: Gui Zhi 3g, Bai Shao 1.5g, Sheng Jiang 1 slice, Da Zao 1 piece, Gan Cao 2g. (Two packets, one per day, taken in three doses)

Three hours after taking the first dose, the episodic colic pain stopped. After two packets, the condition was completely resolved.

CLINICAL INSIGHT

In non-complex diseases, after diagnosing the disease, one can then perform formula pattern diagnosis. From the perspective of Chinese medicine, it was a fairly simple matter to diagnose this child with "running piglet". Then, based on his flushed face, fullness and distention in the abdomen, and palpitations on the navel, I diagnosed him with a Gui Zhi Jia Gui Tang pattern. In performing differential diagnosis of running piglet, one must also consider Ben Tun Tang, which is marked by alternating cold aversion and heat effusion and Ling Gui Zao Gan Tang which has palpitations *below* the navel and no actual running piglet.

Gui Zhi is the main herb that treats running piglet in Gui Zhi Jia Gui Tang. In his chapter on Gui Zhi in *A New Commentary on 'Herbal Patterns'* (重校藥徵), Yōdō Odai (尾台榕堂) states: "Because it treats upward surging, it is indicated in running piglet disease". That said, this understanding runs counter to the modern Chinese medical herbology view of Gui Zhi. In modern Chinese medical herbology, Gui Zhi is seen as a warm, acrid, exterior resolving herb that has an upbearing and floating quality, so how could it possibly treat upward surging? In the 1930s, Lu Yuan-lei commented on this, stating: "In Japan, it is already common knowledge that Gui Zhi treats upward surging, but Chinese medical doctors in China find this ridiculous for some reason." Eighty years later, Gui Zhi's ability to treat upward surging still hasn't been widely recognized in China. In actuality, Gui Zhi's ability to treat upward surging is not some baseless inference on the part of the Japanese, the evidence for this action is readily available in the *Treatise on Cold Damage*. For instance, in line 15 of the Song version it states: "In tàiyáng disease, if a patient develops upward surging of qì after being purged, Gui Zhi Tang can be used. If there is no upward surging, Gui Zhi Tang should not be used." Additionally, in line 17 of the Song version it states, "...In running piglet, when qì surges up from the lower abdomen to the heart...Gui Zhi Jia Gui Tang with an extra 2 liang of Gui Zhi can be used." Thus, students of jīngfāng must remember that "one's way of thinking determines the effectiveness of one's treatment". Students must recognize that jīngfāng and *Inner Canon*-style medicine represent two entirely different modes of thought. Wittgenstein considered using "I'll teach you differences", a line from Shakespeare's *King Lear*, as an epigraph for his *Philosophical Investigations*. This notion of difference in Shakespear was a concept that proved quite an inspiration for Wittgenstein and should for us as well. Learning to spot the asymmetries between jīngfāng and the *Inner Canon* style will help the student of jīngfāng to quickly grasp these concepts of "a generalized theory of disease", "herbal patterns", "formula patterns" and "treating based upon the pattern.

Pediatric Chronic Asthma Treated with Gui Zhi Jia Hou Pu Xing Zi Tang

10 YEARS, FEMALE

CC: Recurrent Asthma

HISTORY: When she was three years old, the patient was initially hospitalized after developing a fever and shortness of breath and was later diagnosed with asthma. Treatment with Western medicine was initially successful in bringing down the fever and resolving the shortness of breath, but the child subsequently developed chronic asthma with frequent episodes that only seemed to get worse with further treatment. At five years old, the patient's family opted to try Chinese medicine. Chinese medical treatment was much more successful—not only did it seem to control episodes more rapidly, it also diminished the frequency of episodes. For the next three to four years, the child did not have a single episode. However, one week ago, after developing a fever and being hospitalized for one week, the asthma returned.

FIRST VISIT: November 8th, 2009

CURRENT:

The patient is emaciated and has a pallid complexion. Her current symptoms were aversion to cold and heat effusion, headache, no sweating, cough and panting with little phlegm, oppression in the chest, and shortness of breath. Her temperature ranged from 37.6–38°C.

PULSE: Floating, rapid, and weak

TONGUE: Pale red with a white coating.

Based upon the above symptoms and signs, I prescribed Gui Zhi Jia Hou Pu Xing Zi Tang. After one packet, the fever abated, and the panting diminished. After three packets, all symptoms resolved.

In September of 2011, she had another asthmatic episode. I treated it using Xiao Chai Hu Tang plus Xiao Xian Xiong Tang.

In 2013, she developed coughing and panting after developing a fever with sweating. I treated it with three packets of Ma Xing Gan Shi Tang.

CLINICAL INSIGHT

Asthma is a common pediatric disease and jīngfāng treatment is often quite effective. Going forward, more research should be done into common patterns of disease and corresponding treatment approaches.

The formula Gui Zhi Hou Pu Xing Zi Tang is not present in the Kang Zhi (康治) version of the *Treatise on Cold Damage* or the *Essential Prescriptions of the Golden Cabinet*. It first appears in the Song dynasty version of the *Treatise on Cold Damage*. The Song dynasty version of the *Treatise on Cold Damage* is based on the *Essential Prescriptions of the Golden Cabinet* and the Kang Zhi version of the *Treatise on Cold Damage*. The *Essential Prescriptions*, in turn, is also based on the Kang Zhi version of the *Treatise on Cold Damage*. This tells us that the work of expanding the science of formula pattern diagnostics and treatment has been developing continuously since the advent of the written word in China and the *Treatise on Cold Damage and Miscellaneous Disease* represents one stage in that process of development.

The pathology corresponding to the Gui Zhi Jia Hou Pu Xing Zi Tang pattern has two distinct etiologies: 1.) Line 18 of the *Treatise* states:

"For those with chronic panting, Gui Zhi Tang plus Hou Pu, Xing Zi is highly indicated." This line describes a patient with a history of asthma for whom a new exterior contraction brought on an asthmatic episode. 2.) Line 43 of the *Treatise* states: "In tàiyáng disease, if the patient develops panting after being purged, this is due to the exterior contraction not being resolved. Gui Zhi Jia Hou Pu Xing Zi Tang is indicated." This patient's asthma developed secondary to exterior cold contraction—they didn't originally have asthma. The etiology and pathological course of these two scenarios is different, but they have the same clinical presentation. As such, according to formula pattern correspondence principle, the same formula should be given in both scenarios.

For patients with fever, coughing, and panting, I often prescribe Gui Zhi Jia Hou Pu Xing Zi Tang, Ma Huang Tang, or Ma Xing Gan Shi Tang. I base my differential diagnosis on the following symptom presentations:

Heat effusion, coughing, panting, aversion to cold, no sweating: Ma Huang Tang

Heat effusion, coughing, panting, aversion to cold, sweating: Gui Zhi Jia Hou Pu Xing Zi Tang (Gui Zhi Jia Hou Pu Xing Zi Tang can also be used to treat patients with the above symptoms and no sweating, but they must have a weaker constitution or a floating, rapid, and weak pulse.

Heat effusion, coughing, panting, sweating, (no aversion to cold): Ma Xing Gan Shi Tang

Pediatric ADHD Treated with Gui Zhi Tang plus Ling Gan Jiang Wei Xin Xia Ren Tang (Phlegm and turbidity obstructing internally type)

MR. LU, 10 YEARS

HISTORY: The patient, the first-born child of his parents, was delivered at full-term and his mother had no illness during pregnancy. For the past five years, the child has suffered from occasional coughing, panting, and diarrhea. Additionally, he was diagnosed with ADHD five years ago. He has trouble focusing at school, is extremely talkative, has trouble sitting still in class, gets nervous about taking tests, and his grades have suffered.

CURRENT: The patient has a thin build and a pallid complexion. He complains of aversion to wind and cold, excessive saliva production, sweats easily with activity, has cold hands and general feeling of cold, constipation, and distention and glomus in the sub-sternum and abdomen.

PULSE: Thin and moderate

TONGUE: Pale with a thin, white, moist coating

ABDOMINAL PALPATION: Flat abdomen, contraction in the rectus abdominis.

DIAGNOSIS: Disharmony of construction and defense, and phlegm and turbidity obstructing internally. Tàiyáng-tàiyīn combination disease.

FORMULA: Gui Zhi Tang plus Ling Gan Jiang Wei Xin Xia Ren Tang: Gui Zhi 6g, Bai Shao 6g, Xing Ren 6g, Ban Xia 6g, Gan Jiang 3g, Zhi Gan Cao 3g, Da Zao 3 pieces, Fu Ling 10g, Wu Wei Zi 5g, Xi Xin 2g. (One packet per day)

After a month of herbs, all symptoms improved, he was able to focus more in class, his appetite increased, and BMs normalized. I continued prescribing the same formula at a reduced dose for three more months, after which his condition completely resolved. In follow-ups over the next two years, he never reported any relapse.

CLINICAL INSIGHT

The *Inner Canon* states: "All wind, falling, and vertigo belong to the liver." Pediatric ADHD can be understood as a kind of wind disease and its disease location is the liver. The patient's aversion to wind, spontaneous sweating and moderate pulse indicated disharmony of construction and defense on the exterior, while his copious saliva, poor appetite, incomplete BMs, and glomus and distention in the sub-sternum and abdomen were indicative of cold phlegm obstructing within. This was a case of interior and exterior combination disease that attacked upward to the heart and liver, leading to a scattering of the spirit and mind, and a tendency towards hyperactivity and logorrhea.

Based upon the patient's thin build, spontaneous sweating, aversion to wind and cold, pallid complexion, and contracted rectus abdominis, I diagnosed him with a Gui Zhi Tang Pattern. Based on his copious saliva, occasional coughing and panting, and pale tongue with white coating, I diagnosed him with a Ling Gan Jiang Wei Xin Xia Ren Tang pattern. By combining these two formulas, I was able to resolve his intractable condition.

TREATISES ON JĪNGFĀNG MEDICINE

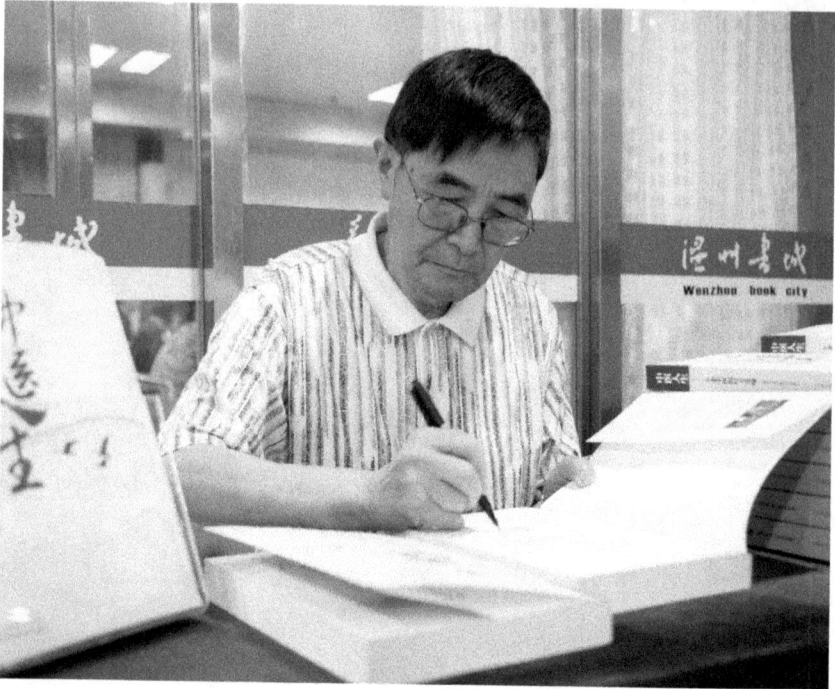

What is Jīngfāng Medicine?

Much importance is placed upon the question of how to define jīngfāng. Some will say that jīngfāng is just the collection of formulas included in the *Treatise on Cold Damage* and the *Essential Prescriptions of the Golden Cabinet,* but I am even more inclined to see jīngfāng as a method of diagnosis and treatment comprised of formula-pattern correspondence and pattern-targeted treatment. In this sense, many post-classical formulas like Er Chen Tang, San Ren Tang, Si Wu Tang, etc. can be considered jīngfāng as long as they are implemented using a jīngfāng methodology. Conversely, if so-called jīngfāng formulas are prescribed on the basis of pathomechanism analysis, then even if the formulas come from the *Treatise on Cold Damage* or the *Essential Prescriptions of the Golden Cabinet,* this still cannot be called jīngfāng.

What Kind of Book is the *Treatise on Cold Damage*?

How should we characterize the *Treatise on Cold Damage*? This is an important question for every student of jīngfāng, myself included. I have been thinking about and researching this question for several decades and, gradually, I've come to my own understanding. The *Treatise on Cold Damage* is a generalized theory of disease. It not only focuses on common characteristics of various disease cohorts, details disease-targeted treatments, and describes how to perform differential diagnosis within disease categories, it also advances a comprehensive approach to disease which takes into account the patient's holistic response to the pathogen, their important symptoms, signs and constitutional characteristics, and then enumerates corresponding formula patterns. This is a fantastic method and one that I've used for several decades now with good results. The more I use this method, the more I see how the *Treatise* presents a generalized theory of disease. As Lu Yuan-lei (陸淵雷) once said, "Chinese medicine can treat disease without having to identify (its material basis). Indeed, Chinese medicine is targeted not at diseases, but at symptoms." This is an extremely insightful statement. If you can apply this statement in your clinical practice, you will be able to reach the level that Xu Ling-tai described as "using jīngfāng in every possible condition".

Jīngfāng Knows No Borders and Can Become an International Medicine

For a long time, people have always thought that one needs a grounding in traditional Chinese Culture and a strong Chinese medical foundation in order to master Chinese medicine. This is not the case with jīngfāng. Jīngfāng diagnosis is based upon direct observation and can be directly applied in clinic via formula-pattern correspondence. This approach does not require so much Chinese medical theory. My German friend Ditmar's experience with studying jīngfāng is a case in point. Ditmar is 55yo this year (in 2018) and has been practicing Chinese medicine for over twenty years. It would be no exaggeration to say he is passionately devoted to jīngfāng medicine. He studied jīngfāng using an English version of the *Treatise on Cold Damage* and treats difficult and intractable diseases using a combination of herbal medicine and acupuncture. In Germany, he has a certain amount of influence and reputation. In recent years, he has come to my clinic for two weeks every year to study and exchange experience. He doesn't speak or read Chinese, so how was he able to develop such a command of jīngfāng? He believes that jīngfāng is a kind of technique or technology that anyone can learn. Ditmar's successful mastery of jīngfāng is a testament to the unique character of jīngfāng described above. As such, I believe that jīngfāng knows no borders and can become an international medicine. I truly believe this and look forward to the day when it becomes a reality.

Chinese Medicine Can Treat Disease Without Having to Identify (Its Material Basis)

An elderly woman who lived near the university suddenly went deaf and was diagnosed with sensorineural hearing loss by Western medicine. A Chinese medicine physician diagnosed her with sudden hearing loss due to liver and kidney dual vacuity. Neither western nor Chinese medicine proved effective in treating her condition, so she came to my clinic. Based upon the patient's small and portly build, pale and dark complexion, aversion to cold, nasal congestion, pale tongue with thin white coating, and a sunken and weak pulse, I diagnosed her with a Ma Huang Fu Zi Xi Xin Tang pattern. Despite her having hypertension, I still insisted on using this formula, prescribing three packets, as it fit her pattern. After just one packet, she recovered her hearing.

FORMULA: Fu Zi 9g, Xi Xin 3g, Ma Huang 6g.

ACUPUNCTURE PROTOCOL: SJ21, SI19, KI3

Three years after I treated the elderly lady, her daughter-in-law sought me out to treat her dacryocystitis. I had never studied ophthalmology and had no understanding of the etiology of dacryocystitis or blepharitis, much less did I know how to differentiate between chronic and acute dacryocystitis. So, I told her that I hadn't treated anything like what she had before, but I could prescribe her something based upon her pulse and symptoms.

I told her, "In ancient times, all diseases were treated with Chinese medicine. Perhaps ancient Chinese medicine didn't have names for all the diseases they encountered, but "Chinese medicine can treat disease without having to identify its material basis". I went on to raise the example of her mother-in-law: I didn't know her mother-in-law had sensorineural hearing loss, but I was still able to resolve her condition by treating her formula pattern.

It was Dr. Lu Yuan-lei who, in his *Medical Treatise of Dr. Lu* (陸氏論醫案集・卷三), said that "Chinese medicine can treat disease without having to identify its material basis". He wrote an easy to understand, engaging, and entertaining chapter on this topic in that book. He said: "Zhang Zhong-jing was able to identify and treat diseases—he was a master physician, not just a run-of-the-mill doctor. But to treat disease, one really needs to identify the pattern, not the disease itself. It is much more difficult to identify a disease than it is a pattern, so if we are just interested on efficacy of treatment, we needn't place much import on the difficult task of identifying disease." I have always kept his theory of Chinese medicine close to my heart and often speak about it with colleagues and patients.

When I first read Dr. Lu Yuan-lei's comments on identifying and treating disease, I found them to be ridiculous and lacking common sense. However, on repeated readings, I came to see that this passage actually spoke to the very essence of Chinese medicine. It seemed to me, that he was saying something that few else were capable of saying or dared to say. The pronouncement of such a statement required not only deep medical wisdom, but also tremendous courage.

Structural Differences Between the
Treatise on Cold Damage and the Inner Canon

In ancient times, there was no separation between science and philosophy. All of the authors who contributed to the *Inner Canon* were essentially concerned with identifying an overarching order, identifying the structure and order hidden beneath the surface of all things, and uncovering the mysterious organizing principle uniting heaven, earth and mankind.

The answers they found are at once simple and profound. However, with the arrival of the *Treatise on Cold Damage*, a major paradigm shift occurred — theoretical concerns like "unity of heaven and man", "five movements and six qì", etc., are replaced with clinical findings and direct observations. This led to a fundamental shift in the understanding, diagnosis, and treatment of disease. With the *Treatise*, experience and observation came to replace metaphysical reasoning and speculation as the primary mode of inquiry. Experience is another means by which humans explore and attain knowledge of their surroundings. Zhang Zhong-jing's *Treatise on Cold Damage* is a perfect example of a combination of experiential observation and logical inquiry. His formula pattern diagnosis and treatment strategy is set within the context of yīn-yáng theory. He took the crystallization of wild thought (pensée sauvage)[15] and combined it with yīn-yáng theory, the most powerful ontological system of the day. Simultaneously, he clearly realized the value of

---

[15] Here, Dr. Lou borrows a term from the structural anthropologist Claude Levi-Strauss. We can think of "wild thought" as a form of cogitation that is not overly conditioned by one system of logic, but rather incorporates various systems and heuristics in a more freeform style. In Dr. Lou's writing, "wild thought" typically refers to early ancient physicians' direct engagement with disease and their creative attempts to unite consistencies and make sense of the emerging order unfolding in their experience. Lou sees jīngfāng medicine as a product of wild thought.

formula-pattern diagnosis and endeavored to preserve the original formula-pattern system of the *Methods of the Classic of Decoction* (湯液經法) within his work.

CASE STUDY EXAMPLES

Case #1

MR. HUANG, 60 YEARS (70KG, 167CM)

Patient has a history of hypertension, hyperlipidemia, and hyperglycemia. His face is flushed, and he has a strong build. He complains of headache, vertigo, neck stiffness, numbness of the limbs, bitterness of the mouth, halitosis, and dry, painful throat. He doesn't drink much water and his BMs are sloppy and incomplete, 2–3 times per day. Urine is scant and yellow.

PULSE: Sunken and strong

TONGUE: Dark red with a greasy and yellow coating

ABDOMINAL PALPATION: The rectus abdominis is strong and thick.

FORMULA: Ge Gen Qin Lian Tang: Ge Gen 60g, Huang Qin 9g, Gan Cao 3g, Huang Lian 9g

After taking fifteen packets, all symptoms noticeably improved. I continued using modifications of this formula over an extended period of time and the patient's symptoms all gradually disappeared.

Case #2

FEMALE, 35 YEARS

CC: Trigeminal Neuralgia (Centered at the ophthalmic nerve)

HISTORY: The patient has a thin build and reports having a poor constitution with a childhood marked by frequent illness. After marrying and having children, her health continued to decline even further. Six months ago, she developed trigeminal neuralgia subsequent to an extended cold with sinusitis and dacryocystitis. Prior to seeking me out for treatment, she had self-medicated with painkillers.

FIRST VISIT: Patient has a dark red complexion and complains of heat vexation, aversion to wind, headache, bitterness in the mouth, nausea, fullness and discomfort in the chest and rib-side, constipation, and irregular periods with scant volume and dark, purple menses.

ABDOMINAL PALPATION: Left and right lower abdomen pain upon pressing and a bind in the lower left abdomen.

DIAGNOSIS: The patient has a clear Xiao Chai Hu Tang plus Tao He Cheng Qi Tang pattern.

FORMULA: Xiao Chai Hu Tang plus Tao He Cheng Qi Tang (Three packets)

On the fourth day, the patient reported that the formula had been ineffective.

The *Treatise on Cold Damage* line 144 states: "If a female patient suffers wind strike and develops alternating heat effusion and cold aversion after seven to eight days after which there is a cessation of menstruation, this is heat entering the blood chamber and the blood will surely congeal.

As such, the patient displays a malaria-like heat effusion pattern. In such cases, Xiao Chai Hu Tang is indicated."

Based upon this line, I decided to give the patient straight Xiao Chai Hu Tang. After three doses, her trigeminal neuralgia markedly improved and the heat effusion, aversion to cold, headache, bitter mouth, nausea, and other shàoyáng symptoms vanished. However, the patient still had a dark red complexion, constipation, and the above abdominal presentation. As such, I pivoted to prescribing seven packets of Tao He Cheng Qi Tang, after which her trigeminal neuralgia continued to improve. Three months later, there had been no relapse of symptoms. The practice of jīngfāng medicine is a bit like orienteering—the practitioner is constantly faced with decisions to make about how to proceed. Even if one practices exactly according to the *Treatise on Cold Damage*, there will often be several different possible methods of treatment in any given pathological presentation. The key to successful treatment is choosing the correct formula pattern or the formula that is most appropriate for assisting the body's resistance to the pathogen.

Case #3

MIDDLE-AGED, FEMALE

CC: Insomnia, Copious Yellow Leukorrhea

The patient is overweight and has a yellow complexion. She complains of bitterness in the mouth and halitosis. Her tongue has a greasy, yellow coating. I diagnosed this as phlegm heat assailing the heart and prescribed Huang Lian Wen Dan Tang. The formula was effective, but after a week, her symptoms returned. Wu Ju-tong noted that "One liang of Ban Xia descends counterflow, whereas two liang of Ban Xia promotes peaceful sleep." This means that Ban Xia needs a higher dose to be effective in treating insomnia. As such, I upped the dose of Ban Xia from 9g to 45g. After two packets, the patient reported a significant improvement in sleep that was further improved with a week of herbs. I told her to suspend treatment and monitor symptoms. The patient did not have any relapses of insomnia until two years later after a fit of anger. Her symptoms were essentially the same as before, so I prescribed the same formula with the same high dose of Ban Xia.

Ban Xia's anti-emetic effect is also dose dependent. In the *Treatise on Cold Damage*, 30g of Ban Xia is used in Chai Hu Gui Zhi Tang to treat "slight nausea or vomiting", whereas in Xiao Chai Hu Tang and Da Chai Hu Tang, 50g of Ban Xia is used to treat "frequent vomiting" and "continuous vomiting" respectively. Clearly, the more severe the nausea or vomiting, the higher the dose of Ban Xia is needed.

The *Treatise on Cold Damage* and the *Yellow Emperor's Inner Canon* are Like Conjoined Twins

Our ancestors likely placed such great emphasis on the diagnosis and treatment of disease either out of sheer practical necessity or because they became captivated by this dynamic process of change between health and disease. Practical necessity and mere interest are not equal concerns. The former is a matter of survival, whereas the latter derives from our ancestor's attempt to understand and analyze the world around them. The former led to jīngfāng medicine, whereas the latter led to the pathomechanism-based lineage of the *Inner Canon*. Because the *Treatise* and the *Inner Canon* are products of the same time period and developed during the same era, they have common themes and language despite having different focuses and different paths of development. These common themes, these intersections, have led to a misunderstanding that has stretched on for two millennia. It was Zhong-jing that organized the hitherto shambolic strands of formula-pattern experiential knowledge into a coherent three-yīn three-yáng system.

The aspects of the *Treatise on Cold Damage* that focus on the dynamic principles of diagnosis and the priority of treatment between root, branch, acute, and chronic pathologies are influenced by the *Inner Canon*. Tōdō Yoshimasu's brazen removal of the three-yīn three-yáng system from the *Treatise* deprived practitioners of a means of classifying pathological presentations and stands as a significant step backward in the development of jīngfāng as a clinical medicine. Faced with complex diseases, the formula-pattern style's only move is to use combinations of formulas to make sure they've "covered all their bases". However, this style of practice lacks an understanding of differentiating between primary and secondary symptoms, acute and chronic presentations, and combination, dragover, and aggravated disease. Without an understanding of these principles, one's clinical efficacy will surely suffer.

Cold Damage Versus the
Inner Canon's "Febrile Disease"

Warm disease is a sub-class of cold damage. Cold damage includes all common exterior febrile disease. This is why in the *"Treatise* on Febrile Disease" in the *Simple Questions* it states, "Damage by cold results in febrile disease" and "so-called 'febrile diseases' are all a form of cold damage".

Quotes from *Inner Canon* authors are interpolated throughout the *Treatise*. For instance, in Line 4 of the Song version it states: "On the first day of cold damage, the pathogen enters tàiyáng. If the pulse is unremarkable, it has not passed into the next channel[16]. If there is nausea, agitation, vexation, and a rapid pulse, it has penetrated into the next channel." Line 5 states: "After two to three days of cold damage, if yángmíng and shàoyáng symptoms haven't surfaced, the pathogen has not passed into the next channel." Line 8 states: "In tàiyáng disease, when headache resolves by itself after seven days, this is because the pathogen has passed through all channels. To prevent the pathogen from passing through the channel sequence again, needle foot yángmíng."

We can prove that the above three lines come from the *Inner Canon* authors of febrile disease theory based upon the following points:

The *Treatise* and the *Inner Canon* list different durations for passage between channels. In the *Inner Canon*, channel passage occurs every day of febrile disease. Thus, it states, "on the first day of febrile disease, the pathogen is in tàiyáng" and "on the second and third days the pathogen is

---

[16] In jīngfāng, we typically refer to 經 as "conformation" to reflect the fact that the pathology is a full-body phenomenon that is not restricted to the channels. The *Inner Canon*, by contrast, centers its theory of febrile disease around the channels. To avoid confusion, I translated all instances of 經 in this passage as "channel", but one should keep in mind that in the *Treatise*, 經 should be understood as conformations.

in yángmíng and shàoyáng respectively". By contrast, in the *Treatise*, the pathogen is thought to stay in tàiyáng for five to six days before channel passage.

The order of channel passage in the *Treatise* and the *Inner Canon* are different. The *Inner Canon* febrile theory authors put yángmíng before shàoyáng, whereas in the *Treatise*, yángmíng comes after shàoyáng. For instance, Da Chai Hu Tang and Chai Hu Jia Mang Xiao Tang patterns would only appear after a Xiao Chai Hu Tang pattern.

The *Treatise* includes statements like "when the patient has suffered from tàiyáng disease for six to seven days", "when the patient has suffered from tàiyáng disease for eight to nine days", "When, after ten or more days of tàiyáng disease, there is channel passage" and "after suffering from shàoyīn disease for two to three days". What do these passages tell us? Zhong-jing is telling us that exterior febrile diseases won't pass through all six channels, three yīn diseases won't always arise after passing through yáng channels, and the pathogen will not necessarily pass through one channel per day.

As noted above, the second half of Line 8 states, "The pathogen has passed through all channels. To prevent the pathogen from passing through the channel sequence again...". This passage draws from the idea of the cyclical nature of channel passage described in the "Treatise on Febrile Disease" and is in stark contrast to the *Treatise*'s idea of channel passage occurring once every six to seven days with the threat of death occurring if the pathogen passes through a number of channels and does not recover. The cyclical channel sequence described in the "Treatise on Febrile Disease" does not accord with clinical reality in the slightest.

The *Inner Canon* is primarily a collection of works by acupuncturists, whereas the *Treatise* is primarily an herbal work. In Line 5, however, it states that the method for stopping the pathogen from channel passage is to needle at the foot yángmíng (source point). It is quite likely that this is a case of the work of an *Inner Canon* acupuncture-based author's work being interpolated into the *Treatise*.

Consider for instance, in the course of treating an exterior febrile disease, a patient who is first diagnosed with typhoid fever, later begins to exhibit malaria-like symptoms followed by dysentery-like symptoms. From the perspective of modern bacteriology, it would be hard to explain how these disparate symptom presentations came about, but from the perspective of the *Treatise*'s channel passage theory, this progression of symptoms can be easily explained. In Lu Yuan-lei's research into channel passage theory in the *Treatise*, he found that there was an inconsistency between the duration of channel passage time and the stage of channel passage.

Cold Damage and Miscellaneous Disease

Cold damage and miscellaneous disease are two large and interrelated categories of illness. Their complicated and complex relationship forms the basic structure of all disease. Cold damage refers to common exterior contraction febrile disease, which often manifests with heat effusion except in rare cases where the person is too weak to mount a febrile response. Patients with miscellaneous disease often do not have heat effusion. Those that do often have a unique main symptomatology. For instance, febrile diseases like meningitis and tetanus both manifest with "tetanic" or spasmodic symptoms while acute pneumonia and acute bronchitis manifest with "cough and counterflow of qì". Additionally, malaria and acute hepatitis are both miscellaneous diseases that exhibit febrile symptoms.

The Order of Chapters in the *Treatise on Cold Damage* Contradicts Clinical Reality

Chinese people have a deep respect for tradition and a reverence for ancient figures, which is why the *Inner Canon* is written as a dialogue between the Yellow Emperor, Qi Bo, and other respectable ancient figures. Zhang Zhong-jing also held this respect for tradition, which is why he kept the order of channel passage in the "Treatise on Febrile Disease", placing yángmíng before shàoyáng. However, in Zhong-jing's actual writing, shàoyáng comes after tàiyáng and before yángmíng, so Chai Hu patterns do not arise after channel passage to yángmíng and are not recorded in the shàoyáng chapter, which is why the shàoyáng chapter appears strangely empty. Zhang Zhong-jing had no choice but to abide by this order, but this also shows how his system is not perfect. Within this ordering, we see the inner struggle that Zhong-jing must have gone through—interesting indeed.

Formula Pattern Diagnosis in the Context of Six-Conformation Diagnosis

The six conformations of the *Treatise on Cold Damage* describe six different "syndromes" and were created to systematize and streamline the process of diagnosis and treatment. What distinguishes the three yáng syndromes from the three yīn syndromes is the disease-resisting strength of the patient, while the three yáng syndromes themselves are differentiated based upon the location of the disease in the body. Tàiyáng disease occurs in the upper part of the body as well as on the surface, yángmíng disease occurs in the interior of the body and below, while shàoyáng disease occurs in the space in between. As for the three yīn, shàoyīn disease occurs when there is exterior contraction febrile disease in patients with weak heart function, tàiyīn disease occurs when there is gastroenteritis in patients with "center cold" and should not be included in the *Treatise on Cold Damage*. Juéyīn is a long-standing mystery and is likely an artifact of the aggregation of various miscellaneous conditions.

Generally, formula pattern diagnosis is conducted within the context of six-conformation diagnosis—this is the most reasonable form of diagnosis. There is an ancient saying that says, "Those who excel at Go ponder the overall trend of the game, while those who do not excel ponder over single pieces."

In the jīngfāng system of diagnosis and treatment, formula pattern identification and treatment are conducted within the context of Zhong-jing's three yīn three yáng system. Formula pattern "states" comprise the essential elements of this system and they exist in logical and pre-determined relationships. What makes the *Treatise* such an enduring text is that it was able to combine the three yīn three yáng structure with formula pattern diagnosis and treatment in one system. One can comprehend the genius of this accomplishment by considering the various formula pattern "states" that Gui Zhi Tang embodies throughout the structure of the three yīn three yáng system. The dynamic, but self-contained, structure of the three yīn three yáng system is what accommodates the predictable and logical dynamics of various formula pattern states and allows for these formula patterns to be utilized in various forms in the process of diagnosis and treatment. The *Treatise on Cold Damage* creates this enormous field of spatial consciousness, inviting the practitioner to enter into the vast gilded chambers of a palace of unrestricted thought.

Jīngfāng medicine does not view formula patterns as isolated entities — it not only attends to the various layers in the structure of any formula pattern, it also focuses on mutual dependence and restriction between patterns, viewing them as an array of sub-systems. Zhongjing saw formula patterns as a complex, symbolic nodal network that derives meaning not from the symptoms themselves, but from relations of symptoms in combination.

Formula pattern correspondence is not a tool — if jīngfāng practitioners wish to utilize formula pattern diagnosis in the treatment of disease, they must consciously accept to operate within the limitations of the formula pattern correspondence system. Adhering to formula pattern correspondence in clinic should be regarded as the primary attainment of the jīngfāng practitioner. Practitioners should seek to embody formula pattern logic to the point that it becomes an instinct. Only when jīngfāng practitioners absorb formula pattern correspondence into their very marrow and allow it to take root in their hearts will jīngfāng medicine gain a solid footing in our society and free our medicine from arbitrary and subjective methods of prescription.[17]

---

[17] Referring to pathomechanism-based diagnosis and treatment.

Shàoyáng-Yángmíng Dragover Disease

In clinic, there are certainly cases in which the shàoyáng disease hasn't completely resolved but the condition already passes partially into yángmíng. Indeed, in the *Treatise* we can see an example of this kind of shàoyáng yángmíng dragover disease in line 229:

"In yángmíng disease when there is tidal heat, sloppy stools, fullness in the chest and rib-side, and urination is normal, Xiao Chai Hu Tang can be used."

In yángmíng disease with tidal heat, there should be hardened stools and frequent urination, but in this case the stools are sloppy and urine is normal—this indicates that yángmíng replete bowel disease has not yet developed. From "fullness in the chest and rib-side" one can further conclude that the pathogen is also lodged in shàoyáng and cannot be dispelled. One the one hand, the yángmíng bowel repletion has yet to develop, on the other the shàoyáng disease has not yet resolved. These two disease conformations can be viewed as existing in a sequential dynamic and, as such, this situation points to a shàoyáng-yángmíng dragover disease.

There are several potential formula patterns that might arise in the context of this shàoyáng-yángmíng dragover disease. Because multiple formula patterns can crop up in this situation, the *Treatise on Cold Damage* Kang Ping version's use of "Chai Hu Tang" is more suitable than the use of "Xiao Chai Hu Tang" mentioned in the Song, Cheng Wu-ji, and Yu Han versions of the Treatise. "Chai Hu Tang" refers to all the various Chai Hu formulas—in shàoyáng-yángmíng dragover disease we can consider using Xiao Chai Hu Tang, Da Chai Hu Tang, and Chai Hu Jia Mang Xiao Tang, etc. As such, the Kang Ping versions use of the term "is indicated" is unsuitable as it fails to communicate that there are several formulas that can be used in this situation. The Song version's use of "can be used" is much more appropriate in this situation. In his *Explanations of the Treatise on Cold Damage*, Keisetsu Ōtsuka combines the essence of the various versions to give this flawless rendering:

"A patient with yángmíng disease has tidal heat, sloppy stools, and frequent urination. If their urination is normal and they have fullness in the chest and rib-side, Chai Hu Tang can be used."

There are several other examples of shàoyáng-yángmíng dragover disease in the *Treatise*, but they're buried deep in the text and require repeated analysis and comparison along with a knowledge of the "exterior before interior" treatment method of dragover disease to discover them.

Case #1

MIDDLE-AGED, FEMALE

CC: Facial Shingles

The patient developed shingles one week ago and subsequent treatments have been unsuccessful. The shingles are extremely painful. Upon diagnosis, I found the patient displayed signs of several patterns including the Gui Zhi Tang pattern, Xiao Chai Hu Tang pattern, and Xiao Xian Xiong Tang pattern. I combined all three formulas and gave three packets. On the third day the patient returned and said the prescription had been ineffective. After much consideration, I concluded that this was most likely a shàoyáng-yángmíng dragover disease. The tàiyáng aspect was clearly a Gui Zhi Tang pattern, while the shàoyáng aspect was comprised of Xiao Chai Hu Tang and Xiao Xian Xiong Tang patterns. I decided to first prescribe three packets of Xiao Chai Hu Tang. After the first day of herbs, the pain dramatically reduced and after three days, the pain basically completely abated. However, the patient still had a Xiao Xian Xiong Tang pattern, so I gave them three packets of Xiao Xian

Xiong Tang, after which the patient's condition completely resolved. (From Ch.22 "Case Studies" in Lou Shao-kun's *A Life Devoted to Chinese Medicine: One Master Physician's Long Engagement with Jīngfāng*).

Takeaway

This was an unexpected learning experience that arose due to the fact that I didn't succeed in treating the case right away. It reminded me that we are always only a hairbreadth away from failure and led me to place great emphasis on the study of combination and dragover disease.

Case #2

ADOLESCENT, FEMALE

The patient has had a chronic cough for one year that has failed to respond to treatment. The cough resulted from bronchitis subsequent to a cold that failed to completely resolve. Based on the patient's chest and rib-side discomfort and fullness, palpitations above the navel, dry mouth, and plum-pit sensation in the throat, I prescribed Chai Hu Gui Zhi Gan Jiang Tang plus Ban Xia Hou Pu Tang for 1 month with little efficacy. Upon closer questioning, I learned that the patient was extremely averse to cold and had a pallid complexion, so I pivoted to Ma Huang Fu Zi Xi Xin Tang. After taking the formula, her body began to regain warmth, her cough subsided, and before long the condition completely resolved. (Ken Fujihara, The Importance of Dragover Disease, Beijing Chinese Medicine University Journal, 1981 (1): 25)

Ken Fujihara's Insights:

Six-conformation diagnosis can also be used in chronic diseases.

The above case is an example of shàoyáng Chai Hu Gui Zhi Gan Jiang Tang and shàoyīn Ma Huang Fu Zi Xi Xin Tang dragover disease. The Ma Huang Fu Zi Xi Xin Tang pattern was latent and wasn't manifested clearly in signs and symptoms. Ogura Shigenari (小仓重成) called these non-manifesting patterns "latent patterns". The Ma Huang Fu Zi Xi Xin Tang pattern was a "latent pattern", which is why Ken Fujihara didn't immediately discover it.

In shàoyáng Chai Hu Gui Zhi Gan Jiang Tang and shàoyīn Ma Huang Fu Zi Xi Xin Tang dragover disease, treatment should proceed from the urgent condition to the background constitutional condition, this is why Ma Huang Fu Zi Xi Xin Tang should have been used first.

Ken Fujihara (1914–1997)

Ken graduated from Chiba Medical University in 1940 with an MD PhD and worked in the university's Ophthalmology Research and Education Department. He also studied under *kampo* physician Okuda Kenzo (奥田謙藏) and established the Chiba University Oriental Medicine Research Association. In 1950, he participated in the establishment of the Society for Oriental Medicine in Japan and later served as a director, chairman, and councilor of that organization. He also served as the medical director of the Fujihara Ophthalmology Hospital, Fujihara Kampo Research Center director, and was active as a *kampo* educator. He enthusiastically promoted medical exchanges between China and Japan and was named an honorary professor at Shanghai University of Chinese Medicine and a visiting professor at Beijing University of Chinese Medicine. Some of his main works included: *Lectures on Kampo Fukushin, Fundamentals of Kampo, Commentary on the 'Categorized Collected Formulas', Kampo Clinical Notes: Treatises, Kampo Clinical Notes: Treatment Strategies.*

Tàiyáng Shàoyín Dragover Disease

Line 91 of the *Treatise on Cold Damage* states: "In cold damage, if the physician purges the patient and they subsequently develop incessant clear-food diarrhea with body pain, one should first urgently save the interior. Later, when the diarrhea has resolved but there is body pain, urgently save the exterior. Save the interior with Si Ni Tang, Save the exterior with Gui Zhi Tang."

Line 372 states: "When there is diarrhea, distention and fullness in the abdomen, and body pain, first warm the interior, then attack the exterior. Warm the interior with Si Ni Tang, attack the exterior with Gui Zhi Tang."

These two lines both describe tàiyáng Gui Zhi Tang formula pattern plus shàoyīn Si Ni Tang formula pattern dragover disease. Because the shàoyīn disease in these cases is urgent and grave, the method used is to first treat the urgent pattern then attend to the mild pattern just as in line 100.

Dragover diseases are often treated with the "first exterior, then interior" method, but applying this method to the situations in lines 91 and 372 would be a kind of inelastic thinking. In the *Treatise*, urgent and severe conditions are treated using the "first severe, then mild" approach. From this, we can see that Zhong-jing had a nimble, dynamic clinical thinking process which was attentive to the specific contradictions of the condition at hand and not encumbered by dogmatic adherence to protocols.

The description of the exterior and interior symptomatology in line 372 is decidedly concise. For new students of the *Treatise*, this concise language can be difficult. The *Treatise* has a unique lexicon—in line 372, "abdominal fullness and distention" signifies the patient is vacuous. If the patient had a replete condition, Zhong-jing would just use "abdominal fullness". With the one exception of its inclusion in the principal symptoms for tàiyīn disease, abdominal fullness is always a sign of repletion, be it in cold or heat patterns. Thus, from the mention of "fullness and distention in the abdomen" in line 372, we can infer the patient also has other vacuity symptoms and signs such as "comfort with heat or massage, lack of abdominal springiness, and a weak and deficient vacuity pulse".

When studying the *Treatise*, students must be extremely attentive to the subtleties of language used, otherwise they will easily fall prey to misunderstanding. For instance, "heat effusion" refers exclusively to the form of heat expressed in tàiyáng disease and is always accompanied by "aversion to cold". The form of heat expressed in shàoyáng and yángmíng disease is not called "heat effusion". Furthermore, the word "stomach" in the *Treatise* actually refers to the intestines. The actual stomach is called "below the heart" or "the sub-sternum" in Zhong-jing's lexicon. Lastly, the terms "vomiting counterflow" (嘔逆) and "eructation counterflow" (吐逆) do not refer to the same symptom. "Vomiting counterflow" describes a feeling of churning in the stomach with nausea, while "eructation counterflow" refers to burping, etc.

The term "heat effusion" appears throughout the *Treatise* and typically requires comparison with concomitant symptoms to arrive at a diagnosis. Shàoyáng disease also has heat effusion, but it's typically expressed as "alternating aversion to cold and heat effusion" or "vomiting with heat effusion. Only in line 165 describing the Da Chai Hu Tang pattern does it state, "cold damage with heat effusion". The forms of heat expression in yángmíng disease include "body heat", "heat", "tidal heat", "late afternoon tidal heat", etc.

The Three Urgent Purging Patterns in the Shàoyīn Chapter Are Interpolations of *Inner Canon* "Treatise on Febrile Disease" Authors

Lectures on the Treatise on Cold Damage[18] contains a distillation of the insights and experiences of the great commentators throughout the ages. It is a very reasonable and authoritative volume on the *Treatise*. Most commentators throughout the ages have concluded that the three urgent purging patterns in the shàoyīn chapter all represent conditions in which shàoyīn is pivoting out into yángmíng and developing due to the pathogen stagnating in the middle and developing into a bowel disease. Everyone says this is a "shàoyīn" condition, but they still adhere to a formula-pattern correspondence principle and prescribe Cheng Qi Tang based on a yángmíng bowel repletion diagnosis.

Experienced doctors use an approach that focuses on "treating the pattern", "formula pattern correspondence" and "setting aside empty names to attend to the actual substance" to achieve effective diagnosis and treatment in shàoyīn urgent purging patterns. However, the average physician might be thrown off by the apparent contradiction between the name and the actual condition and might even end up "depleting vacuity patients and supplementing replete patients".

---

[18] This refers to the Li Pei-sheng (李培生) version published in 2008 by Shanghai Science and Technology Press (上海科学技术出版社).

Differential Diagnosis of Tàiyáng Exterior Patterns Is Very Important

Differential diagnosis of exterior patterns is a common topic in Chinese medicine, but successfully treating exterior conditions is no simple matter. In the *Treatise on Cold Damage*, exterior patterns are primarily found in the tàiyáng chapter. Zhong-jing's analysis of exterior patterns is extremely precise and exacting—indeed, he devotes nearly half of his treatise to this subject. Why does Zhong-jing spend so much time on exterior patterns? Lu Yuan-lei's explanation was that tàiyáng disease is the most difficult to understand, so Zhong-jing had to go to great lengths to clarify his understanding. He likened this to splitting bamboo: At first, great strength is needed to penetrate the fibrous outer layer, but once the knife slices through, the bamboo can be split with the slightest effort.

The great physicians of every age have always based their evaluation of their students by their ability to treat exterior conditions. There is a story about a famous Shanghai physician that sent his son off to study with another colleague when he was in his early teens. The colleague had the child split his time between reading the classics and following him in clinic. Later on, he had his son study with another colleague for a year before sending him off to a Japanese medical school. Five years later, after his son graduated from medical school, the Shanghai physician first had his son follow him for one year before letting him have his own rotation in their clinic. This would allow the son to be able to go to his father for questions whenever he came upon a difficult case. He also stipulated that to reassure his patients, for cases involving high fever, tuberculosis, drum distension (late-stage hepatic disease), and tumors, the father would be the primary physician. In this way, the physician's son gradually improved his clinical skills over the course of two years.

One afternoon when the father had traveled out of town to see a patient, another patient with a high fever for two weeks arrived at the clinic. The son had no choice but to take the patient and he quickly diagnosed him with a Ma Huang Tang Pattern. He decocted the formula for him at the clinic and had the patient take it right away and stay in the clinic for observation. After two hours, the patient developed a slight sweat, his fever slightly abated, and he began having alternating cold aversion and heat effusion with bitterness in the mouth, nausea, chest oppression, and a pale tongue with yellow, greasy coating. The young doctor prescribed two packets of Chai Qin Qing Dan Tang[19].

When his father returned, the young doctor related how he had treated the patient and awaited his father's response. The father was quiet for quite some time, then, suddenly, a smile crept across his face, and he clapped his hand on the table, saying: "You won't go hungry now!" What he meant is that his child could now practice medicine independently. He then invited the entire family as well as the two colleagues that had tutored his son to participate in a lavish banquet at a big Shanghai restaurant to celebrate that his son "wouldn't go hungry".

The son was a bit puzzled. He wondered to himself: "Why was there no banquet or celebration after I completed my studies with my two teachers or after I graduated from medical school? Why the big celebration just because I prescribed a dose of Ma Huang Tang? Isn't Ma Huang Tang a basic formula that we all learn early on in our training?" The father knew full well what his son was thinking and said to him: "Son, remember this: knowing something in theory doesn't mean you really understand it. And understanding something doesn't mean you know how to use it in clinic. You can only be considered to have gained a basic level of competence once you've truly grasped formula pattern correspondence, and only then will you "not go hungry". "Not going hungry" means being able to support yourself by utilizing your skills."

The father continued in a hushed tone: "Ma Huang Tang is part of the spirit of Chinese medicine. When you have enthusiasm for Chinese

---

[19] Composed of Chai Hu, Huang Qin, Ban Xia, Chen Pi, Gan Cao, Zhu Ru. So, like a combination of Xiao Chai Hu Tang plus Wen Dan Tang.

medicine, it will treat you well, but if you have a falling out, if you lose your enthusiasm for the clinic, that spirit will quietly depart. Son, I hope that the spirit of Chinese medicine will stay with you throughout your life."

I'm not sure if this is a true story, but it had a big impact on me all the same. It made me constantly worry that the spirit of Chinese medicine would leave me and pushed me to continue reading commentaries and other works on the *Treatise on Cold Damage* to find traces of this elusive spirit. For decades, I've used Ma Huang and Gui Zhi formulas to successfully treat infertility, central serous chorioretinopathy, HIVD, and other interior diseases. Through this process, I've gradually come to get a sense of how to use these exterior-resolving herbs. Whether one is treating an exterior or an interior condition, the first order of business is to ascertain whether there is exterior contraction. If there are any signs of exterior contraction, I almost always first resolve the exterior. Through my clinical experience, I've come to realize why exterior contraction is the very first of the ten questions.

I once treated my student's aunt who had suffered from trigeminal neuralgia for seven years. During flares, she would experience excruciating pain in her upper and lower teeth and temples. She had previously pulled three teeth in an effort to relieve the pain. The pain was bearable during the day, but at night it would intensify to the point where she couldn't sleep. When she came to my clinic, she presented with an exterior pattern consisting of aversion to wind, heat vexation, lack of sweating, and a floating and tight pulse. Based on these symptoms and signs, I prescribed one packet of Ma Huang Tang. Early the next morning, shortly after I woke up, I heard a banging on the door and upon opening it, I saw the woman with the trigeminal neuralgia standing there on my stoop. To my shock, she said she hadn't slept a wink the entire previous night.

"How is the pain in your teeth?" I asked.

"Strangely, I haven't had any pain in my teeth and temples today." She replied.

"When did you take the medicine?" I asked her.

"I took the first dose at 8pm and the second dose at 11pm." She said.

"You waited the right time in between doses, but you started taking it too late. You probably were experiencing a side effect from the stimulatory effect of Ma Huang."

Based upon her symptoms, I prescribed her 3 doses of Si Ni San and let blood at EX-HN5. I told her that if she had any relapse of symptoms, she could come back to my clinic any time. She lived on an island off the coast of Wenzhou, so I never heard from her after that. One year later, when I asked my student how she was doing, he said she never had a relapse of symptoms.

This case helped me realize that miscellaneous diseases often also will have an element of exterior contraction. If there is an element of exterior contraction and it isn't addressed, it might be hard to resolve the condition because exterior contraction is a whole-body pathology, and its influence can be much more powerful than local pathologies.

Identifying exterior contraction should be a basic skill possessed by all Chinese doctors, but to put it bluntly, the number of doctors that do not possess this skill nowadays is by no means small. This is a very depressing reality! Indeed, identifying exterior contraction is not always an easy task. To demonstrate the difficulty of identifying exterior contraction, I want to share the story of Hui Tie-qiao (惲鐵樵) abandoning his career in literature for medicine.

In 1911–12, Hui Tie-qiao worked first as an editor and translator at a commercial press and later as the head editor at a monthly literary magazine. He placed great importance on the structure, organization, and literary style of the writings he edited and would often say, "Good literature should have an enduring and perennial quality". He put little stock in the fame or standing of authors—his only standard was quality, and he placed particular emphasis on cultivating young talent. When Lu Xun submitted his first novel *Nostalgia* to the monthly literary magazine under the pseudonym Zhou Chuo, Hui Tie-qiao was the only editor to recognize its literary value and placed it as the first story in that month's edition. He also wrote an extremely enthusiastic and positive review of the piece for his readers, a move that left a deep impression on the young

Lu Xun (鲁迅). Some twenty years later, Lu Xun mentioned Hui in a letter to cultural worker Yang Qi-yun. Though his tenure at the magazine had little to do with medicine, during his career as an editor Hui was exposed to Western medicine and developed literary skills that would help him when he published Chinese medicine books later in life.

Just as Hui Tie-qiao's career was taking off, he lost three sons to various febrile diseases in the course of two years. Hui had some understanding of medicine and believed he knew how his sons should be treated, but due to his lack of experience, he was afraid to prescribe them herbs himself. However, when he tried to discuss his children's cases with doctors, they were unreceptive. To his dismay, he had no recourse but to put his children's lives in these doctors' hands and hope for the best. After this experience, he realized he couldn't rely on other doctors anymore and made up his mind to study medicine. He devoted himself to deep study of the *Treatise* and also arranged to follow a master jīngfāng physician named Wang Lian-shi. (汪莲石) One year later, his fourth-born son fell ill and presented with heat effusion, aversion to cold, lack of sweating, and panting. This was clearly a tàiyáng cold damage Ma Huang Tang pattern. However, despite the fact that the doctor he called on to treat his son was familiar with the *Treatise*, he didn't dare use cold damage formulas and prescribed him warm disease formulas consisting of Dou Chi, Shan Zhi, Dou Juan, Sang Ye, Ju Hua, Xing Ren, Lian Qiao, and other herbs. After taking these formulas, his son's panting and heat effusion only worsened.

Hui Tie-qiao couldn't sleep and spent the whole night pacing back and forth, pondering over his child's case, unable to make up his mind. But by the morning he had decided, he would prescribe his child one dose of Ma Huang Tang. He told his wife: "Three of our sons have died of cold damage, now Jin-hui is sick, and the doctor says there's nothing he can do. Better for him to die after taking my prescription than to sit here with our arms folded and wait for his eventual death." His wife didn't respond, and he immediately went to prepare the decoction. After one packet, his son's skin became damp and his panting slightly subsided.

After another dose, he broke a sweat, his fever abated, and the panting completely resolved.

After this successful case, Hui became even more convinced of the power of jīngfāng formulas and devoted himself to the study of the classics. When family or friends got sick, he would often treat them with positive results. In one particular instance, a colleague's son had yīn pattern cold damage and even the most famous doctors in Shanghai were unable to reverse his condition, but Dr. Hui stabilized his condition with just one dose of Si Ni Tang. The family was incredibly grateful and wrote a thank you note in a Shanghai newspaper saying: "If your child is sick don't worry, just go see Hui Tie-qiao." After that, he had more patients coming in every day and eventually he decided to quit his literary career and devote himself to medicine in 1920. He quickly rose to become one of the most famous doctors in Shanghai.

I was absolutely amazed when I first heard this story and had so many questions. At the time, of course, I could only ponder over those questions by myself. Given Hui Tie-qiao's social status and the fact that he had some knowledge of medicine at the time, I imagine that he was able to get some of the best doctors in Shanghai to treat his son. They would have had a much deeper understanding of pathomechanisms and diagnosis, and their experience would have far outstripped Dr. Hui. This might have been one of the first prescriptions Dr. Hui had ever written, so why was it that it was so much more effective than the others? There is only one answer: whether knowingly or unknowingly, Hui Tie-qiao was using formula-pattern diagnosis while the other doctors were still caught up in warm disease style pathomechanism diagnosis. Despite being the most famous doctors in Shanghai in the 1920s, they didn't have any real skill. They still hadn't really learned how to identify and differentially diagnosis exterior contraction.

The Difficulty of Diagnosing Exterior Contraction

"Fundamental principles are the most important aspect of any science and the most basic of the fundamental principles are the most important of all the principles." In Chinese medicine, exterior patterns can certainly be counted among the most basic of principles. However, identifying and diagnosing exterior patterns is no easy task. The following example should make this quite clear.

A teacher from my former work unit once sought me out to ask me an interesting question. He said: "My son often catches colds and whenever he develops a fever, I get into an argument with my wife. Why, you ask? My wife is a nurse in a local hospital, and according to Western medicine protocol, if a child has a fever over 39°C, the child's shirt should be unbuttoned to help abate the fever. However, I always disagree, arguing that from my own experience with colds, I always feel aversion to wind and cold and want to be covered with blankets as much as possible. Me and my wife hold opposite views, so we always end up getting into fights. Who do you think is right?

I responded, saying: "This is a very important question in the field of medicine. You and your wife are both right in some ways and wrong in others. When a child has a fever, one must analyze the other concomitant symptoms in the manner of Chinese medical pattern differentiation. Only after conducting pattern differentiation can you determine who is right. Your wife's symptom-based treatment approach is certainly the preferred method of treatment in Western medicine. Chinese doctors might also use this method in combination with acupuncture and herbs if there is an internal heat pattern.

The teacher couldn't quite grasp my explanation and responded: "Could you just tell me in "plain English" in which situation I would be right and which situation my wife would be right?"

I replied, saying: "If when your child has a fever, he also presents with aversion to cold, your method would be correct. If the patient doesn't feel aversion to cold or wind when he has a fever, then your wife's approach is better."

He seemed a bit confused and asked: "How do we know if the child is averse to cold?"

I said: "It's fairly easy to identify aversion to cold. If his skin has goosebumps in the presence of cold, that's a cold aversion response."

He nodded with satisfaction.

I continued: "If there is aversion to cold, then no matter how high the fever is, Chinese medicine classifies the condition as "exterior cold contraction" and uses acrid warm herbs to resolve the exterior. Simultaneously, the patient should also be kept warm to induce sweating. If the patient does not have aversion to cold and wind in the presence of fever, they have an internal heat pattern. In such cases, they would need heat-clearing fire-draining herbs, and their clothes should be unbuttoned to allow heat to diffuse."

He thought for a moment and then asked: "If he has a fever and just a slight aversion to cold how would the disease be classified according to Chinese medicine?"

I was impressed by his thorough questioning and responded: "This would be an externally contracted wind-heat pattern. Chinese medicine would use Yin Qiao San. In such cases, he shouldn't be wearing heavy clothes or be under heavy blankets and should make sure to drink enough water." He nodded happily and left satisfied.

Examples of Complex Presentations
in Tàiyáng Exterior Patterns

A physician cannot easily predict if a patient's tàiyáng disease will pass into yángmíng. Also, due to countless unpredictable factors, the disease can also pass into the three yīn. As such, when presented with tàiyáng disease, the physician must first treat the tàiyáng disease. When using warm, acrid herbs to resolve the exterior in tàiyáng disease, if the physician can first warn the patient that the formula might cause the disease to pivot into yángmíng, they won't be as worried when it happens. This is much different than trying to explain to the patient what happened after the fact. What's important is to have an understanding of how the disease might evolve over time so you are not surprised and overwhelmed by the patient's presentation.

Disease progression in the tàiyáng stage of external febrile disease can be very complex—in some cases the exterior cold pattern will resolve upon sweating after using acrid, warm herbs, in some cases the fever will only slightly abate after sweating and in other cases the fever will not only not abate after sweating, but it might also increase to a higher temperature. Below are two example cases detailing this complexity.

March 9th, 1975: A seven-year-old girl with a strong constitution suddenly developed a high fever of 40°C with coughing and panting five days ago. She was diagnosed with bronchitis and treated using standard western protocols with little success. Her family asked that she be treated with Chinese medicine.

CURRENT: The patient complains of heat effusion, aversion to cold, transparent rhinorrhea, headache, panting, cough and lack of sweating. Her

245

pulse is tight and rapid (110bpm), and her tongue coating is thin and white. This is wind-cold exterior contraction. In tàiyáng disease, if the defense qì cannot effuse outwards, it may transform into heat and pass inward. The appropriate treatment method is to resolve the exterior, induce sweating, effuse the lung, and calm panting using Ma Huang Tang.

Ma Huang 4.5g, Gui Zhi 3g, Xing Ren 7.5g, Sheng Gan Cao 3g.

Three hours after taking the first dose, the patient developed a slight sweat, her temperature returned to normal, and all symptoms resolved.

August 10th, 1975: A three-year-old female patient developed continuous high fever, drowsiness and desire to sleep, and rigidity of the nape of the neck four days ago and was diagnosed with possible Japanese encephalitis by a local hospital. Her parents refused a lumbar puncture, so the diagnosis could not be confirmed. She was treated with western and Chinese medicine, but her condition worsened, and her family eventually decided to bring her to my clinic for treatment. The child was somnolent, displayed nausea with occasional vomiting, had a fever of 41°C, her forehead was hot to the touch, and her feet were cold. Her pulse was floating and rapid (130bpm). Her parents tried to bring her temperature down by placing a cold towel on her forehead and fanning her with fans, but upon inspection, the child had goosebumps, a clear sign of aversion to cold. The patient had a white and glossy tongue coating, rigidity in the neck, and a positive Kernig's sign. Based upon the patient's neck rigidity, heat effusion, aversion to cold, lack of sweating, floating and rapid pulse, white and glossy tongue coating, and occasional nausea, I prescribed Ge Gen Jia Ban Xia Tang to resolve the exterior, induce sweating, upbear fluid, and course the collaterals.

Ge Gen 9g, Ma Huang 4.5g, Gui Zhi 3g, Bai Shao 6g, Sheng Gan Cao 3g, Da Zao 3 pieces, Sheng Jiang 6g.

Additionally, I told her parents that high fever in exterior contraction is the body's natural response to the pathogen and there was no need to use other methods to bring the fever down. Two hours after taking the first dose, she broke a sweat and her temperature dropped to 38°C, she complained of thirst, and her nausea and vomiting ceased. After fanning her with a large fan, I noted that she no longer displayed goosebumps. She was still somnolent, had aversion to wearing heavy clothes or using blankets, her urine had gone from clear to yellow, she had not had a bowel movement that day, and her pulse had changed to surging and large. Clearly, her condition had pivoted into the yángmíng stage, and as the Qing dynasty researcher of yángmíng disease Lu Mao-xiu stated, there are no fatal conditions in yángmíng. As such, I knew the most dangerous stage of her condition had passed. I then prescribed Bai Hu Jia Ren Shen Tang. After two doses, her fever completely abated, and she had no lingering symptoms.

Why Tàiyáng Exterior Patterns
are Difficult to Diagnose

The Negative Impact of Pathomechanism Theory on Diagnosis of
Exterior Patterns

As is well known, an "exterior pattern," "表證" refers to a symptom
pathology consisting of aversion to wind and cold, heat effusion, headache and a floating pulse which occurs due to the effect of a pathogenic
evil that has penetrated into the superficial layer of the body. In Chinese
medicine, exterior patterns are further differentiated into an exterior
cold syndrome and an exterior heat syndrome based upon symptoms
and signs. Differential diagnosis of exterior cold and exterior heat syndromes should be performed based upon symptom patterns as opposed
to etiology of disease. Unfortunately, the warm disease school excessively
emphasized the importance of etiology, a development that had a negative impact on the thinking process of Chinese medical physicians. They
came to hold the erroneous belief that all infectious disease is warm disease, that heat effusion is the primary symptom of warm disease, and
warm evil damaging yīn is the primary pathomechanism. As a result, it
became common practice to diagnose infectious diseases with exterior
presentations as "exterior heat", infectious diseases with interior presentations as "interior heat", at the qì level as "qì heat" and so on. In this
way they came to associate the pathomechanism of various symptoms
for the pathomechanism of the disease as a whole. Following a certain
deterministic logic of external causes, they turned a pathomechanism,
which is a sufficient condition for the genesis of a pathology, into a necessary condition for determining the nature of the disease. This fallacy
continued to spread and has had a very negative impact on the diagnosis
of exterior contraction.

CHINESE MEDICINE TEXTBOOKS

For at least half a century, Chinese medicine textbooks have stated that exterior cold patterns will have a floating and tight or floating and moderate pulse, while exterior heat patterns will have a floating and rapid pulse. There are two very basic mistakes with this assertion. First, when performing differential diagnosis, a comparison must be made between two similar qualities. However, in the above statement, a floating and tight or moderate pulse is compared with a floating and rapid pulse, but these are two different qualities. The former refers to the tightness of the pulse, while the latter refers to the speed of the pulse. There is no way to compare the tension in a pulse to the speed of the pulse because they are two different qualities (rapid versus slow would be an appropriate comparison). Such a comparison has no differential diagnostic value. To use a rural colloquial phrase, "Mom and dad say 'heaven', while the son-in-law says 'earth'."[20] Second, in severe exterior cold patterns, the patient's temperature will rise and naturally their pulse will become rapid. As such, Ma Huang Tang patterns can present with floating, tight and rapid pulses, while Gui Zhi Tang patterns can present with floating, moderate, and rapid pulses. Indeed, we can see examples of this throughout the *Treatise*. Due to this erroneous statement in Chinese medicine textbooks, many physicians mistakenly diagnose exterior cold patterns as exterior heat patterns. This is why many doctors are incapable of using warm, acrid herbs.

MISTAKING THE NORMAL PROGRESSION OF DISEASE FOR IATROGENESIS

Exterior cold patterns often completely resolve after using warm, acrid herbs to induce sweating and resolve the exterior, but it is also common for the patient's temperature to increase after using herbs. Some physicians will erroneously believe that the increase in temperature is due to

---

[20] Meaning, one has nothing to do with the other.

the warm, acrid herbs and be less likely to use them as a result. Lu Mao-xiu wrote a fantastic commentary on the normal progression of exterior contraction. He argued that after correctly using warm, acrid herbs to resolve the exterior in an exterior cold pattern, it is a good sign if the remaining cold evil transforms into heat and pivots into a yángmíng presentation. The real worry in external contraction is yīn damage, yáng collapse, and pivoting into the three yīn. Thermometers weren't available in the Qing dynasty, but most anyone with clinical experience will be aware that temperatures usually run higher in the yángmíng stage than in tàiyáng. Lu Mao-xiu devoted himself to the study of yángmíng disease and he eventually concluded that yángmíng is like when a criminal gets cornered in an alley—they might make a big fuss, but there is nowhere for them to go. As long as treatment is timely and formulas are applied correctly, the patient will surely recover. As such, he famously said, "there are no fatalities in yángmíng."

In some cases, patients might develop nose bleeds after taking warm, acrid, exterior-resolving formulas. Zhong-jing wrote about this long ago and later authors began calling it "red sweat"—it's a sign of recovery. However, patients and their families sometimes mistakenly believe normal changes in the progression of a disease like nose bleeds and escalating temperatures are a sign that the physician has made a mistake. They may believe that the physician mistakenly used a warm, acrid formula on an exterior heat pattern, and the above changes are evidence of their error.

Incorrect Criteria for Differential Diagnosis

The symptom and sign criteria for the differential diagnosis of exterior versus interior conditions is clear, but the criteria for differential diagnosis of exterior heat patterns versus exterior cold patterns is more controversial. In febrile diseases, especially in high fever, certain heat-related symptoms like high temperature, rapid pulse, dry mouth, light yellow urine etc. are not particularly useful in the differential diagnosis between exterior cold and exterior heat. The most important symptom in the differential diagnosis of exterior patterns is aversion to cold and wind. "Slight aversion to cold or no aversion to cold" in exterior heat patterns demonstrates that the "exterior" aspect of the exterior heat pattern is already weakening, and the condition is already moving towards the first stage of interior heat with just the slightest bit of exterior contraction remaining. This is why the acrid, cool exterior resolving formula Yin Qiao San consists mainly of heat-clearing herbs with just a few acrid, dispersing herbs. The main acrid, dispersing herb is the warm, acrid herb Jing Jie. Because of this confusion regarding the criteria for differential diagnosis in exterior patterns combined with the negative influence wrought by pathomechanism-based thinking, many have difficulty identifying the primary symptoms that help differentiate the exterior pattern.

Treating the Common Cold is Chinese Medicine's First Clinical Lesson

Treating "the common cold" should be a basic skill that all Chinese medicine practitioners possess, but, at the risk of sounding offensive, there is no small number of Chinese medicine practitioners that are incapable of treating the common cold. This might be hard to believe, but it is the unfortunate truth.

With regard to the treatment of exterior contraction, the *Inner Canon* states: "For exterior effusion, one should not shirk from using warm herbs and for interior purging one should not shirk from cold herbs." During and before the Jin (晋) and Tang dynasties the primary method for treating exterior patterns was resolving the exterior with warm, acrid herbs. During the Jin (金) and Yuan dynasties, the physician Liu He-jian (劉河間) promoted the use of acrid, cool, sweet and cold herbs to resolve the exterior, trailblazing a new path in the treatment of exterior patterns. His student, Zhang Zi-he (張子和), took a middle road, stating: "In cold damage disease use Zhong-jing's approach and in febrile disease use He-jian's approach." During the Ming and Qing dynasties, warm disease split off from the Cold Damage school and became an independent system. Their approach which used acrid, cool herbs in exterior contraction and bitter cold herbs in latent pathogen disease gradually became systematized. Since the late Qing dynasty and with the spread of warm disease theory, preference for acrid, cool herbs and disdain for acrid, warm herbs became a kind of fashion among practitioners. In an effort to rectify the misguided beliefs of the majority of their contemporaries, cold damage school practitioners ended up going a bit overboard in their correctives. Lu Mao-xiu, for instance, claimed that tàiyáng disease only has an exterior cold pattern and exterior warm patterns are all actually yángmíng disease. Lu Yuan-lei continued to propagate this idea. In his essay, "Warm Disease is Not an Independent Category of Disease Outside of Cold Damage" he states: "Ever since I began studying with my teacher, I have never used Yin Qiao or Sang Ju to treat so-called warm disease and I've never seen any cases of abnormal passage to the pericardium as a result. In the rare situation I did see so-called pericardium patterns, it was typically after a patient had taken Yin Qiao or Sang Ju. As such, I have concluded that abnormal passage to the pericardium results from using acrid cool herbs in exterior contraction. Doctors nowadays will make a show of predicting passage into the pericardium after prescribing acrid, cool formulas. Patients find this amazing and the doctors are even amazed at their own predictive capacities." (From *The Medical Cases and Treatises of Dr. Lu, Volume 3*) These are incisive statements, but they are an exaggeration and slightly biased.

The cold damage school is not alone in recommending warm, acrid, exterior-resolving formulas in the early stage of a cold—Gui Zhi Tang is also the first formula listed in the warm disease school classic *Detailed Analysis of Warm Disease* (溫病條辨) by Wu Ju-tong (吳鞠通). The fourth line in that book states: "In the early stage of tàiyīn wind warmth, warm heat, pestilence warmth, and winter warmth with aversion to wind and cold, Gui Zhi Tang is indicated. If there is only heat effusion, thirst and aversion to cold, the acrid, cool, balanced formula Yin Qiao San is indicated. Wu Ju-tong additionally stated: "There is cold aversion in cold damage because tàiyáng is the conformation of cold water and rules the exterior, but there is also cold aversion in warm disease because the lung is connected with the skin and body hair and also rules the exterior." In his *Clinical Guidance and Case Studies* (臨證指南醫案), Ye Tian-shi (葉天士), a noted warm disease specialist, also records many cases of using warm and acrid herbs to resolve the exterior. This clearly demonstrates that while the cold damage and warm disease schools represent different angles on the question of exterior contraction, their approaches are united by the objective reality of the clinical encounter.

In summary, we must have a holistic and complete understanding of exterior contraction. Clinical reality shows us time and again that no matter what type of exterior evil is involved in the exterior contraction, the presentation in the early stage of the disease will almost always involve aversion to wind and cold, necessitating the use of warm and acrid exterior resolving herbs. This is why the major physicians from all the lineages of the Japanese *kampo* tradition, including Keisetsu Ōtsuka, Dōmei Yakazu, Ken Fujihara, Tōtarō Shimizu (清水藤太郎) and Kazuo Tatsuno (龍野一雄) all agree that Gui Zhi Tang and Ge Gen Tang are the first-choice formulas in the early stage of exterior contraction and acute infectious disease. Indeed, they often recommend Ge Gen Tang as an important "home medicine cabinet" formula for the early stage of exterior contraction.

In Formula Pattern Diagnosis, It is Not Always Necessary to Determine a Pathomechanism Based on Symptoms

Let me start this essay by recollecting an experience I had that inspired me to study jīngfāng and become a doctor.

During the Great Chinese Famine, I returned to the countryside with my father to participate in agricultural work and also began my study of acupuncture under the physician Dr. He Huang-miao (何黄淼). I happened to come upon a copy of Lu Yuan-lei's medical treatises during that time, and it was from that book that I learned about formula-pattern diagnosis and the importance of the *Treatise on Cold Damage*. After pouring over Dr. Lu's impassioned treatises, I became a loyal "long-distance acolyte" of his and began studying the works of Zhong-jing in earnest. Over the course of the next three years, I treated many of my fellow villagers with acupuncture, but I still hadn't prescribed a single formula and was extremely eager to do so.

A young farmer in my work unit ate too many eggs and rice dumplings during the Dragon Festival and developed diarrhea, vomiting, and abdominal pain. He was diagnosed with acute gastroenteritis by a local Western medicine hospital and his condition partially resolved with treatment. However, he still complained of stomach distention, excessive eructation, and sloppy stools for several months. He was treated by several Chinese doctors who all diagnosed him with food damage and gave abductive dispersion and transforming accumulations formulas, but these prescriptions were not only ineffective, they actually exacerbated his issues. In three months, he lost over 10kg and eventually came to me seeking treatment. After intake, I concluded that he had a Ban Xia Xie Xin Tang formula pattern based upon his substernal glomus, vomiting and nausea, and borborygmus with sloppy stools. Based on the fact that he also had insomnia and occasional canker sores, I prescribed Gan Cao Xie Xin Tang.

At the time, I was young and confident, and I was sure that the formula would be effective because the patient's symptoms perfectly matched the formula pattern. In diagnosing this patient, I used formula pattern diagnosis — understanding of the pathomechanism was not requisite for diagnosis. I was inspired to use this approach after seeing how Zhong-jing used Gui Zhi Hou Pu Xing Zi Tang. Regardless of whether the patient had chronic asthma or had been purged with herbs, as long as their presentation fit the Gui Zhi Hou Pu Xing Zi Tang formula pattern, Zhong-jing would use the formula. After prescribing the formula, I resolved to myself that if the formula was ineffective, I would stop studying Chinese medicine. But after taking three packets, the patient reported that all symptoms had noticeably improved. I was absolutely overjoyed and knew that I had finally found a proper path of study. As long as I put in effort to master jīngfāng, I would eventually come to grasp the very essence of Chinese medicine. I took this to be the first milestone in my career as a Chinese doctor.

The *Inner Canon* represents an inchoate stage of Chinese medicine development centered around pathomechanism-based treatment; thus, it states: "All diseases arise from wind, cold, summer-heat, damp, dryness, and fire." In this stage of development, the common form of treatment was suppression of the pathogen, as in "Treat cold with heat and heat with cold". In clinical practice, this method of treatment is largely ineffective — in many cases, new symptoms crop up before the original condition has even been resolved. Even if it does allow temporary relief, there is often relapse. Through clinical failure, Chinese physicians realized that overly emphasizing external sources of disease was a narrow and restricted approach to treatment and more focus should be put on the body's response to the pathogen. As such, *Simple Questions* Ch.74 advises: "Pay close attention to the pathomechanism and understand how each symptom reflects dysfunction in the organs and bowels." Zhong-jing was a clinical practitioner and his six-conformation system arose from his clinical practice. He had little use for patho-mechanisms and focused mainly on formula-pattern correspondence, establishing the formula pattern diagnostic system.

Warm disease theory developed and expanded Zhong-jing's system, but their practice of naming diseases based upon pathomechanisms like "spring warmth", "winter warmth", etc., is regrettable and led to a lot of confusion in later generations. There is a story regarding this issue that will help elucidate my point.

In 1943, while Dr. Wan You-sheng (萬右生) was still a medical stu-dent, his mother developed a fever and was diagnosed with possible typhoid fever. The renowned doctor that Dr. Wan asked to treat his mother diagnosed her with damp warmth and prescribed heat-clear-ing and damp transforming herbs, however, her condition continued to worsen. She appeared somnolent, drowsy, fatigued, and had a poor appetite. She had a thick white tongue coating, and her pulse was rapid. Dr. Wan suggested using a Ren Shen method, but the renowned doctor disagreed, saying, "supplementation is not allowed in damp warmth". He only agreed to remove some of the bitter, cold herbs from the for-mula. On the second day, the patient's fever suddenly dropped, her limbs became cold, and she curled up in a ball. These were classic symptoms of a shàoyīn severe illness. It was only then that the renowned doctor thought to use Si Ni Tang plus Ren Shen, but it was too late—she per-ished before the formula was decocted.

This case demonstrates how disease pathomechanism is not a dependable basis for diagnosis. Even when used by a renowned doctor, such a methodology can still be faulty. In clinical practice, formula pattern diagnosis is a simple and unadorned method that even a new student can learn. However, we must be careful not to go to the other extreme and become like the Japanese Koho (古方) lineage with their "orthodox" formula-pattern approach[21]. Pathomechanisms reflect the basic contradiction of disease, while formula pattern reflects the

---

[21] In this context, "Orthodox" just means, these *kampo* schools practice formula-pattern diagnosis more strictly, with little to no consideration of mechanisms.

primary contradiction[22] in the body's dynamic process of response to the pathogen. Zhong-jing's diagnostic method prioritizes formula-pattern correspondence, but that does not mean that pathomechanisms should be entirely abandoned.

I once had a patient who presented with full-body joint pain, redness, swelling, heat, and pain in the joints of the lower limbs, dry mouth, bitterness in the mouth, desire to drink cold fluids, rapid pulse, and a thick, yellow tongue coating. This seemed like a clear damp-heat Cang Zhu Bai Hu Tang formula pattern, but the formula was ineffective. Indeed, it made the patient's symptoms worse. Upon closer questioning, I learned the patient developed the condition after getting caught in a downpour. I reasoned that the patient had a hidden cold-damp pathomechanism that was driving the disease progression and prescribed 5 packets of Wu Ji San. The patient reported a significant reduction in symptoms that was completely resolved after another 10 packets.

It was for this reason that Dr. Wan You-sheng began researching post-classical formulas late in life. Likewise, Dr. Liu Du-zhou advocated using a combination of jīngfāng and post-classical formulas in his later years. They were clearly driven to these decisions through their own cumulative clinical experience, of which only they know the details.

In summary, I believe that in most cases, it is not necessary to consider the pathomechanism in the process of diagnosis, but I do admit that in certain special cases, pathomechanism thinking may need to assume a guiding role.

---

[22] Dr. Lou is again borrowing terminology from Mao Tse-tung's *On Contradiction*. We can understand basic contradiction here to mean something like a generalized understanding of the cause of disease. Primary contradiction, by contrast, means the main site and scene of conflict, ostensibly between upright and evil qi. The nature of this conflict will change throughout the course of the disease, which is why Dr. Lou calls it "dynamic".

"Identifying the Pathomechanism and Establishing the Treatment Method" and "Prescribing Formulas and Individual Herbs" Are Two Stages of One Diagnostic Process

Separating "Identifying the Pathomechanism and Establishing the Treatment Method" (理法) from "Prescribing Formulas and individual Herbs" (方藥) has led to this current moment where theory and clinical practice have become out of synch. Perhaps I'm overstating the problem a little. Formula-pattern diagnosis and pathomechanism-based diagnosis are slightly different methods of diagnosis. There are similarities and differences between them—we needn't touch upon the similarities as it is the differences which are really worthy of further analysis. To be honest, in the last two millenia, very few Chinese have bothered to perform a serious comparison of these two systems. In fact, only the Japanese seem to have really put much thought into this question. Thus, in Zhang Tai-yan's (章太炎) preface to Lu Yuan-lei's *A Modern Commentary on the Treatise on Cold Damage* (傷寒論今釋·序言), Zhang stated: "If Zhong-jing were alive today, he would no doubt lament that his art was only truly being practiced in the east (Japan)". We should take some time to learn from the Japanese, to engage in this process of step-by-step comparison, differentiation, contrasting and analysis, and we must apply all this in clinic, setting forth on a new, rigorous and modern path of Chinese medical discourse. Indeed, it is truly a shame that there are still some who have not attempted to engage with *kampo*'s formula-pattern diagnosis approach, have yet to understand the strengths and weaknesses of formula pattern and herb pattern diagnosis, have yet to master the skill of formula pattern diagnosis in the treatment of illness, and have never experienced the joy of an instantaneous result achieved after correctly diagnosing a formula pattern.

In Chinese medicine, there are two main kinds of theory: there is "guiding theory", which includes ideas like yīn-yáng, eight principles and six conformations, and then there is explanatory theory. In Zhongjing's *Treatise on Cold Damage*, the primary method is to "observe the pulse and symptoms, identify the site of counterflow and disorder and treat according to the pattern"—this is a kind of formula pattern diagnosis and treatment within the structure of six-conformation theory. "Identify the site of counterflow and disorder" refers to a mechanism-based diagnosis, while "treat according to the pattern" refers to a formula and herb pattern diagnosis. Nowadays, many Chinese medicine physicians believe that proper diagnosis and treatment requires strictly adhering to the "identifying principles, devising methods, choosing a formula and prescribing medicinals" protocol, but in reality, there is another diagnostic process that proceeds in precisely the opposite order (from medicinals, to formulas, to methods to principles). Of course, the guiding theory in that kind of diagnosis is yīn-yáng theory.

Formula pattern diagnosis derives from experience and the direct, visceral reality of clinic. Mechanism-based diagnosis is based on a rational or logical approach. Without logic, there is no Chinese medical theory—all that remains are the building blocks of individual experience embodied in the formulas recorded in books like *Prescriptions Worth a Thousand Gold* and *Essential Secrets from the External Official Library* (外台秘要).

The Negative Influence of Pathomechanism Theory on Chinese Medicine

As everyone knows, an exterior pattern refers to a collection of symptoms and signs including aversion to wind, aversion to cold, heat effusion, headache, and a floating pulse that arise due to evil acting upon the surface of the body during the early stages of exterior contraction. These exterior patterns can further be classified as exterior cold or exterior heat depending upon the patient's symptom and sign presentation. The basis for the differential diagnosis of exterior cold and exterior heat should be symptoms and signs and not a pathomechanism, but the warm disease school overly emphasized the importance of disease pathomechanisms, a development which had a negative effect on the thinking process of Chinese physicians. In turn, it became common for physicians to mistakenly believe that all infectious diseases were warm diseases, that heat effusion was a symptom exclusive to warm disease, and that the primary mechanism of infectious disease was warm evil damaging yīn. As such, it became established doctrine that infectious diseases manifesting in the exterior must be exterior heat, while infectious disease of the interior must be interior heat etc. The transmission of this erroneous theory had a negative impact on physicians' diagnosis of exterior patterns.

The negative influence that pathomechanism theory has had on Chinese medical diagnosis should be taken very seriously. The 20th century physician and China Academy of Chinese Medical Sciences distinguished researcher Lu Guang-shen (陸廣莘) has conducted extensive research on this subject. The formula pattern and herbal pattern diagnostic system of the *Treatise on Cold Damage* is grounded in a theory of internal causes of disease. Indeed, already in the *Inner Canon* we see a gradual shift in theory from the external cause determinism of "all

diseases arise from wind, cold, summer heat, damp, dryness, and fire"
to the interior cause determinism of "all diseases arise from an imbalance of qì and blood." Here we are discussing what later generations
have called "discerning the cause of disease through analysis of symptoms". This is a process of deduction from the body's reaction to disease
in which the physician arrives at an understanding of the nature of the
exterior contraction of external evils via an analysis of the body's multi-
faceted reaction to them. Yet, throughout the course of the development
of Chinese medicine, the search for the correct understanding of pathogens and exterior assailants has never ceased, and it reached a fever
pitch in the Ming and Qing dynasties. Were pathogens mainly cold or
warm, did they enter through the nose and mouth or the skin, what distinguished new from latent pathogens, where did the latent pathogens
lodge, which qì and yùn govern which seasons, etc., all these questions
put an excessive emphasis on the environmental, climatic, and pathogenic causes of disease. The true vitality and theoretical value of Chinese
medicine lies not in questions of environmental, climatic, and pathogenic causes of disease, but in an obsessive focus on the various external
manifestations of the body's disease fighting systems in the dynamic
process of health and illness.

An Insight on Formula Pattern Diagnosis

In previous chapters, I have recounted how a successful clinical experience set me off on my path of practice and study of jīngfāng medicine, but the sheen of that initial success soon wore off. Subsequently, I found that in many cases, I got inconsistent results using formula pattern diagnosis. This caused me to realize that diagnosing purely based off of formula pattern is not enough.

For instance, take one case I had of a 22-year-old male with Hepatitis B. Based on the patient's weak constitution, substernal glomus and hardness, vomiting and nausea, sloppy stools, canker sores, insomnia, and yellow urine, I prescribed Gan Cao Xie Xin Tang, but this formula proved ineffective. I went from bright-eyed enthusiasm to utter confusion and bewilderment. What made me most anxious was that I had no idea why the treatment was ineffective. Only years later and after much study did I slowly come to understand that a formula pattern consists of much more than a tidy set of symptoms—it is a much broader and more expansive form of nosology that can include information about the patient's constitution and a spectrum of western diseases. As such, I began to call this expanded version a "formula pattern condition". Based upon this understanding of formula pattern, I might have diagnosed the above patient with a "Chai Hu Gui Zhi Gan Jiang Tang formula pattern condition". For a patient with a sturdy, strong constitution suffering from gall bladder stones and presenting with substernal glomus and hardness, vomiting and nausea, sloppy stools, canker sores, insomnia, and yellow urine, I'd be likely to diagnose this as a "Da Chai Hu Tang formula pattern condition". If the patient has an endomorphic constitution suffering from diabetes and presenting with substernal glomus and hardness, vomiting and nausea, sloppy stools, canker sores, insomnia, and yellow urine, I'd be likely to diagnose this as a "Ge Gen Qin Lian Jia Ban Xia Tang formula pattern condition".

"Formula pattern condition" diagnosis is an approach with a lot of promise because it conforms to a certain logic. Even in complex cases, the way the body responds to disease always still conforms to predictable principles and patterns, principles which the formula pattern conditions embody.

Formula Pattern Diagnosis and the "De-*Inner Canonization*" of the *Treatise on Cold Damage*

The formula pattern diagnostic system advanced in the *Treatise* is so extraordinary and so mystifying that if it hadn't actually developed out of the "pre-jīngfāng medicine" of the pre-Han era, it would be hard to fathom the existence of such a simple but effective diagnostic approach.

The power of formula pattern diagnosis is beyond the reckoning of human imagination, it exceeds our every expectation. The fact that the ancient Chinese seemingly hit upon this system out of the pure coincidence of clinical experimentation and empirical rigor and were able to preserve it and develop it into something great is a true achievement. Formula pattern diagnosis is likely the final result of a protracted process of struggle between man and disease. Through experimentation, rectification, emulation and summarization, they found that only by adhering to certain principles could they preserve the health of the large majority people and reduce or eliminate the great suffering which disease inflicts. Formula pattern diagnosis and treatment allowed people to take command of an otherwise disparate and vast accumulation of experiential knowledge and deploy it to achieve an unimaginably high level of therapeutic efficacy. Once this system developed and matured, it was no longer necessary for people to seek out a common understanding of all things as people in ancient times had pursued, because all their disparate and vast knowledge and technology could now be channeled through this magical system to achieve effective treatment of disease. At first, people were not aware that this system was better than any of the others — they didn't know that it would markedly improve their diagnostic and treatment abilities. However, through a process of selection and elimination throughout the long durée of Chinese history, our ancestors finally were able to develop this system and effectively transmit it through the generations. *The Divine Farmer's Materia Medica* (神農本草經) and *Yi Yin's Classic of Herbal Decoction* (湯液經法) present the grand achievements of a long and gradual process of accumulation and development of clinical experience. If not for these records of that extended process of countless clinical encounters, experimentation, rectification and imitation embodied by the *Materia Medica* and *Yi Yin's Classic*, Zhong-jing would have been like an artist without a muse. Zhong-jing ingeniously integrated and improved upon the achievements of pre-jīng-fāng medicine. Armed with a single-minded determination forged from devastating family tragedies wrought by the wars and epidemics of his day, he conducted extensive clinical observation, studied and modified formulas from previous generations of jīngfāng practitioners, adjusted how herbs and formulas were combined, and after a protracted process of research, observation and clinical experimentation, finally completed his *Treatise on Cold Damage and Miscellaneous Disease*. As the title of this book subtly suggests, the primary goal of the *Treatise on Cold Damage and Miscellaneous Disease* was to establish an approach to diagnosis and treatment that could be used for all disease.

Tōdō Yoshimasu's formula pattern orthodoxy was a revolutionary moment in the history of interpretations of the *Treatise*. This entirely novel conceptualization was like a bolt from the blue that illuminated the very essence of the *Treatise* and his discovery of formula pattern correspondence ushered in a new era of Japanese *kampo* medicine. His historic contribution was to reframe the relationship between theory and experience in traditional Chinese medicine. Traditionally, theory was superimposed onto experience and they were cast in mutual opposition. In the *Treatise*, however, there is no binary opposition between theory and experience, they form an inseparable whole. Yoshimasu resolved the opposition between theory and experience, allowing them to be subtly integrated and mutually inclusive. In his system, there was no pure experience and no pure theory.

Tōdō Yoshimasu's work is distinguished by his singular focus on elucidating the symptoms of formula patterns. It is for this reason that he was strongly opposed to the consideration of mechanisms in the process of diagnosis and treatment. This approach reflects the tendency of the Japanese to prize empiricism over theory, so it was no surprise that the approach gradually gained acceptance within the Japanese traditional medicine community and later rose to prominence through the Koho lineage, which is now the dominant school within Japanese *kampo*. Certain Japanese scholars have said that the emergence of the Koho lineage triggered a renaissance in Japanese traditional medicine, while others criticized the lineage's emphasis on experience as a step backward for medicine. But if it were really a step backward, why did Tōdō Yoshimasu and other practitioners of the Koho lineage achieve such laudable clinical outcomes? Yamamoto Iwao (山本嚴) weighed in, saying: "The emergence of the Koho Lineage was not a step backward, in fact, it ushered in the scientization of traditional medicine."

The jīngfāng school has never held a dominant position in the Chinese medical world of China in the 2000 years since the writing of the *Treatise*. Formula pattern correspondence was the result of a process of natural selection that occurred in the ancient Chinese medical world—it is a standard of practice in jīngfāng medicine, but during the Song and Yuan dynasties, prominent medical scholars and physicians edited and amended the *Treatise* using ideas from the *Inner Canon*. This led to the emergence of a series of master physicians of the "mechanism" or *Inner Canon* school like Zhang Jing-yue, Ye Tian-shi and Wang Meng-ying who were adept at adapting and implementing jīngfāng formulas for their own purposes. It also spurred the maturation and development of the mechanism school of *Treatise* studies. From the perspective of the jīngfāng school, this was a process of *"Inner Canonization"* of the *Treatise*. Since that time, true formula pattern diagnosis jīngfāng medicine ceased to exist in China.

There were problems, however, with Tōdō Yoshimasu's approach. For instance, he abandoned *Inner Canon* yīn-yáng theory despite the fact that it was the prevailing theoretical model of the Han Dynasty, a model that

Zhong-jing himself also embraced. Without the structuring of a holistic, overarching system like yīn-yáng or six-conformation theory, formula pattern diagnosis lacks a guiding principle and proves insufficient on its own. Though formula patterns are meaningful in and of themselves, yīn-yáng and six-conformation theory invest them with a kind of formal logic, this is why modern jīngfāng medicine cannot abandon theory and also why the theory it embraces should not derive from the *Inner Canon* mechanism school. That being said, if not for Yoshimasu's promulgation of formula pattern orthodoxy and his advocacy to remove *Inner Canon* theory from analysis of the *Treatise*, modern jīngfāng medicine would still be wandering around in the dark.

Formula pattern orthodoxy was a profound and extreme position, but it breathed new life into the practice of formula pattern diagnosis, expanded the range of its influence in the medical community, and allowed it to gain wide acceptance and use in practice. While it can be argued that the formula pattern orthodoxy approach was a kind of overcorrection, if not for this overcorrection, jīngfāng would never have broken free from the spell of *Inner Canon* mechanism theory and returned to a diagnosis and treatment system truly centered around the *Treatise*. To try to remedy the "overcorrection" of formula pattern orthodoxy and improve its lack of structure and organization, Yoshimasu's student developed "qì-blood-water theory". Later on, there were also people like Kitetsu Naitō (内藤希哲) who advocated for a return to *Inner Canon*-style analysis. During this period, Kotokei Nakajin, (中神琴溪) Shinsai Nakanishi (中西深斎) and other Koho school practitioners took up a middle position, arguing for an approach that balanced theory and formula pattern practice. This latter approach was later espoused by many of the greats of the twentieth century, including Yumoto Kyushin, Keisetsu Ōtsuka and Dōmei Yakazu.

From the perspective of historical materialism, it is really no surprise that the call to remove *Inner Canon* theory from analysis of the *Treatise* initially came from Japan. In the early twentieth century, metaphysics and mechanistic materialism first arrived in Asia when the Japanese looked to the west for help while modernizing and industrializing their economy. It was through the influence of this new scientific mindset of mechanistic materialism that Tōdō Yoshimasu came to develop his ideas of about "de-*Inner Canonization*" and led to this "overcorrection" of the complete severing of the connection between the *Treatise* and the *Inner Canon*. Metaphysics and mechanistic materialism have many inadequacies, but these theoretical systems represented an indispensable phase in the evolution of human epistemology. In the *Grundrisse*, Karl Marx states, "Human anatomy contains a key to the anatomy of the ape. The intimations of higher development among the subordinate animal species, however, can be understood only after the higher development is already known." This idea, which is a kind of paraphrasing of Marx's "reflection theory", helps us understand why "de-*Inner Canonization*" took place in Japan as opposed to China.

Tōdō Yoshimasu was without a doubt correct to say that Chinese medical theory is abstract, where he went wrong was when he conflated "abstract" with "abstruse" or "obscure". After all, yīn-yáng and six-conformation theory represent precise and tangible categories that guide diagnosis and treatment in real-world clinical settings.

After entering into the world of jīngfāng through the lens of Japanese *kampo* medicine, it is important to read through the original language of the *Treatise* several times. Nothing can deliver that deep, refreshing breath of medical and intellectual engagement quite like reading the text itself. The process of analyzing and interpreting the *Treatise* should be marked by dialogue, communication, give and take—it should involve arriving at a consensus or common understanding. However, this process was, in some ways, thwarted by the tendency of commentators throughout history to invoke *Inner Canon* theory in their interpretations of the *Treatise*. As Lu Yuan-lei said in his *Modern Commentary on the Treatise on Cold Damage*, "Commentators writing after the Jin and Yuan dynasties became entrenched in their single-minded focus on the *Inner Canon* and nothing would shake their devotion. They elevated isolated phrases and ideas (from the *Inner Canon*) to the status of foundational principles and ran wild with their empty statements while neglecting to discuss actual clinical efficacy." Indeed, reading commentaries of the treatise from after the Jin and Yuan dynasties will only make practitioners more confused and will lead to ideological splits such that, "Every person (will have) their own version of the *Treatise*". Even Dōmei Yakazu's *Commentary on the Treatise on Cold Damage* fell prey to this issue.

The *Treatise* has its limitations, it's not an encyclopedia with rigid, precise definitions and we should not view Zhang Zhong-jing as some kind of prophet on par with Moses. Instead, we must approach the text from our modern viewpoint and reinterpret the texts and probe them for new insights. That is to say, modern jīngfāng scholars and practitioners must create a new space and a new language to inhabit the space between the *Treatise* and modern Chinese medicine and not just take the *Treatise* "as it is" with no qualification. The development of formula pattern orthodoxy and the ensuing birth of the Japanese Koho school is an example of this kind of innovation. Likewise, even though Yumoto Kyūshin had a profound respect for the *Treatise*, he didn't practice jīng-fāng or interpret the *Treatise* "to the letter"—indeed, some of his greatest achievements involved innovative new insights. Mori Dōhaku (森道伯) developed his "therapeutic constitutional theory" from Zhong-jing's writings; his strength was in independent thinking and synergistic analysis. In summary, the *kampo* masters all incorporated a profound amount of new knowledge into their studies and ultimately, it was by dint of their own clinical and intellectual labors that they established their legacies in the annals of the jīngfāng lineage, and not through passively parroting Zhong-jing and his texts.

Due to various issues with the structure of the text of the *Treatise*, new Chinese medicine students will often be confused and put off by what they perceive to be discontinuities between and within lines of the book and might even feel like they are reading a corrupted or incomplete text. When combined with the fact that the book was written some two millennia ago, many will find it extremely difficult to truly understand the *Treatise*. However, by mastering three basic concepts, Zhong-jing's meaning and intent will gradually become clear. These three concepts are: 1.) Six-conformation diagnosis and their passage and transmutation, 2.) Formula pattern correspondence, 3.) Categories of formulas and their mutual relations. If you can focus on and grasp these three concepts, you will have a much easier time studying the *Treatise*.

Ultimately, the *Treatise* is a text made up of sentences and words and the various connections, transitions, dynamics and developments occurring between them. There are many differences between the concepts represented in this text and actual clinical reality. An overarching or general system will inevitably contain some amount of ambiguity because to achieve specificity and precision, some amount of universality must be sacrificed. This is a paradox that Zhong-jing must have grappled with while writing the *Treatise*. In order to capture certain general principles and patterns of disease, Zhong-jing dispensed with certain specific details. As a result, the lines of the *Treatise* inevitably contain a degree of ambiguity and vagueness. This is perhaps why many commentators throughout the ages have noted that students must also give credence to the "implicit" content of the *Treatise*, that which Zhong-jing may have omitted but which can be inferred through context. Due to the use of this sub-textual implied meaning in ancient Chinese literature, it would be quite difficult to truly understand the *Treatise* by focusing on the literal language of the text itself. This implicit layer of the *Treatise* is both an important layer of meaning for us to explore and a barrier to studying and understanding the text. On this matter, Chen Bo-tan (陳伯壇) had an insightful comment: "When interpreting Zhong-jing's original writing, don't worry about whether certain lines are out of place or if the language as written is sensible to the modern ear and don't concern yourself with the various disagreements of interpretation between various schools, just ground your understanding in clinical reality. Zhong-jing's work at once teaches us to find meaning in the text's lacuna while also finding the embodiment of his words in the physical manifestations of patients. Indeed, all of Zhong-jing's writing can already be found hidden within the twelve channels of our patients. To lose one's patients is to lose Zhong-jing." Japanese *kampo* practitioners have put a lot of effort into this analysis and we would be remiss to dismiss the fruits of their research. This form of inquiry invites an opportunity to delve deeper into the *Treatise* and uncover the hidden mysteries awaiting within.

Formula patterns inferred from implicit context in the *Treatise* do not derive their authority from the text itself, but rather from "personal conviction". Personal conviction is not about self-righteous justification, but rather about trying to find one's voice through practice and experience. In my own clinical experience, I've found that each time we treat someone successfully using Zhong-jing's formula pattern diagnosis, we gain a deeper understanding of the *Treatise* and, simultaneously, our "personal conviction" will strengthen. This is not unlike an analogy Hegel once made to elucidate the idea of the creative impulse — he described how when a boy throws a stone into a lake, the billowing ripples from the stone on the face of the water inspire a sense of his own strength growing inside of him, of a heightening of his visual acuity, of an awakening of his spiritual sensitivity and of a subtle vitality, suppleness and flow welling forth from within. That is to say, that the act of throwing that stone produced not only the outward image of that billowing ripple, but also engendered a new sense of self within the boy. Though this inward dynamic was invisible to the eye, it could be clearly and tangibly felt. As long as the physician focuses on the changes in their patient before and after treatment and pays close attention to the subtle dynamics of each case as they unfold, their sensitivity, insight and powers of observation will all improve. This fact can be born out time and again in our every clinical encounter. Clinical practice is thus a process by which we can come to an understanding of the *Treatise*, it is a kind of embodiment of Zhong-jing's will and intentionality. Clinical practice is and forever will be the forebear of theory and knowledge.

Reflections on a Liu Du-zhou
Post-Partum Diarrhea Case

Liu Du-zhou's achievements in the realm of Chinese medicine scholarship are unquestionable, but his journey of clinical development proceeded along a truly windy and indirect path. For the greater part of his life, he was a proponent of the mechanism school and only came to his approach of "identifying the key pattern" in his later years—how many years he must have wasted in the process. In the following post-partum diarrhea case, we can see the schism beginning to form in his clinical thought process.

LIU DU-ZHOU'S CASE OF TREATING ONE MS. CUI

Ms. Cui developed diarrhea after delivery of her first child and was subsequently diagnosed with spleen vacuity and treated with warm supplementing herbs, but this treatment proved ineffective. Her tongue was crimson red with a thin, yellow coating and her pulse was sunken and slightly slippery. On her first visit, I misdiagnosed her as having Juéyīn heat dampness diarrhea based on her having diarrhea plus thirst, and prescribed Bai Tou Weng Tang. On her third visit she complained of coughing, insomnia, lower limb edema, inhibited urine, BMs 3–4 times per day, and thirst with a desire to drink. After pondering over her symptom presentation for a while, I suddenly realized that this was neither a case of vacuity or dampness but was rather a Zhu Ling Tang formula pattern, which typically consists of coughing, vomiting, vexation, and thirst. I prescribed her five packets of Zhu Ling Tang, after which her diarrhea ceased, her urine was disinhibited, and all other symptoms resolved.

In his commentary on the case, Liu Du-zhou remarked: "This was a case of yīn vacuity with mutual binding of heat and water seeping into the intestines and causing diarrhea. As such, I used the yīn-supplementing, heat-clearing and water-disinhibiting formula Zhu Ling Tang."

This case serves as a record of the contradictory nature of Liu Du-zhou's clinical thinking process. In the first visit, he used a mechanism-based approach to diagnose the patient with Juéyīn heat dampness diarrhea and prescribed Bai Tou Weng Tang with poor results. After much thought, he made a sudden realization and pivoted to a different clinical logic, opting to frame the patient's case in terms of formula pattern diagnosis. He saw that the patient's cough, thirst, and insomnia (perhaps likened to vexation) was comparable to line 319: "In shàoyīn disease, when there is diarrhea for 6–7 days, cough, vomiting, thirst, vexation, and insomnia, Zhu Ling Tang is indicated." Unsurprisingly, once he identified her symptoms as being consistent with the Zhu Ling Tang formula pattern, he immediately attained good results. I found it perplexing, however, that in his commentary on the case, he once again returned to a mechanism-based analysis in which he discusses "mutual binding of water and heat seeping into the intestines".

Later on, Liu's thinking about this case seemed to evolve. In a report entitled "The Key to Jīngfāng is Identifying the Key Symptom Pattern" which Liu Du-zhou delivered at a China-Japan *Treatise on Cold Damage* Symposium held in Beijing in October of 1981, he provided this commentary on the case: "Upon seeing the patient had diarrhea with thirst I diagnosed her with Juéyīn diarrhea and prescribed Bai Tou Weng Tang with poor results. On her next visit, she complained of insomnia, cough, and lower leg edema. I then asked her about urine output, and she said her urine was yellow and inhibited. After performing a thorough intake and meditating for some time on the case, I finally realized that this was a Zhu Ling Tang formula pattern. As line 319 states: "In shàoyīn disease, when there is diarrhea for 6–7 days, cough, vomiting, thirst, vexation, and insomnia, Zhu Ling Tang is indicated." This presentation corresponded quite closely to the patient's inhibited urine, diarrhea, lower limb edema, and insomnia. As such, I prescribed the following formula:

Zhu ling 10g, Fu Ling 10, Ze Xie 10, Hua Shi 10, E Jiao 10 (dissolve). After taking five packets, her urine was disinhibited, her diarrhea resolved, and all other symptoms also resolved. This case demonstrates that treatment will be highly impaired if one does not identify the key symptom pattern — once the key symptom pattern *is* identified, the condition often rapidly resolves. However, it is not always such an easy matter to identify the key pattern. Oftentimes one must endure multiple setbacks and detours before arriving at the correct diagnosis…I believe that "identifying the key symptom pattern" expands the treatment range of jīngfāng formulas, arms practitioners with a new form of skill and knowledge, and takes diagnosis to new soaring heights. Identifying the key symptom pattern is what it means to practice jīngfāng."

He only acknowledges that identifying the key symptom pattern "expands the range of application of jīngfāng…etc." but stops short of embracing it as a primary mode of practice. Dr. Liu would clearly have been aware that mechanism-based diagnosis and "identifying the key symptom pattern" represent two starkly different forms of clinical thinking, but he ultimately was unable to recognize this schism in his own thinking and passed it over, leaving the contradiction unresolved. The successive emergence of mechanism-based diagnosis, Liu Du-zhou's "identifying the key symptom pattern" and finally, Huang Huang's "formula pattern diagnosis" represents a kind of historical reversion to a clinical thinking process more in line with that of the *Treatise*.

Your Conceptual Model Will Dictate
Your Clinical Success

I have learned firsthand through sometimes painful and bitter experiences that the most important thing for a student is not what they've read, but what they haven't read. If you read everything, your clinical efficacy will be at most passable, unless you're a genius. So, the guiding philosophy of Chinese medical educators is very important. Huang Huang said it well: "Conceptual models dictate clinical success."

Abdominal Palpation is Critical for Identifying the Key Symptom Pattern

Let me start with a successful case of mine from the 1970s. During that time, I was working as a teacher in a private elementary school in a small town in Wenzhou. During my free time, I would provide acupuncture and herbal treatments to residents of the surrounding communities and had built up something of a reputation. On July 4th, 1975, a doctor from the village commune brought her father in to see me. His name was Pan De-fa and he was a highly intelligent farmer that served as the director of the communes work unit. His chief complaint was right shoulder pain. He was fairly well-off, so he had the money to treat the condition aggressively; he had seen everyone from top-flight doctors at major hospitals to folk doctors in the countryside. They all diagnosed him with frozen shoulder or what is colloquially called "middle-age shoulder" (五十肩). Chinese doctors see frozen shoulder as a kind of impediment disease caused by phlegm, stagnant blood, dampness and heat congesting in the channels. Having suffered from the condition for over year, he had naturally already tried nearly everything—poultices, pills, granules, decoctions, massage, acupuncture, bloodletting, cupping—but nothing had worked, and had perhaps even made things worse. He was at the point where he could barely work and had essentially left the work unit to fend for themselves. When he arrived at my place for treatment, he complained of right shoulder pain, reduced mobility, inability to lift his arm or carry heavy things and increased pain at night that interfered with sleep. Upon closer inspection, I found he had some atrophy in his right arm and was hypersensitive to pain. Additionally, he complained of heaviness in the head, bitter mouth, poor appetite, yellow urine and constipation. His pulse was rough, and his tongue was dark red with a yellow, sticky coating—signs of that phlegm, stagnant blood, dampness and heat congesting in the channels pattern mentioned above. Looking back through his medical record, it seemed to me that most of the other physicians had treated him correctly according to a mechanism-based diagnosis and treatment model, but results had been lacking and most believed it to be an intractable and anomalous condition.

I approached diagnosis from a key symptom pattern perspective. I had the patient lie on their back and began performing abdominal palpation. I found that the patient had pain upon pressing in the sub-sternum and had a knot with pain in the lower left abdomen that would radiate pain to the inguinal area upon deep pressure. Based upon these findings, I diagnosed him with a Xiao Xian Xiong Tang plus Tao He Cheng Qi Tang pattern. Insofar as these two formulas in combination could clear phlegm heat and undo blood stagnation, the prescription was consistent with the mechanism-based diagnosis. After taking three packets, the patient returned with a smile on his face and said he had passed copious turbid, fetid stools. After passing those stools, he said he felt much more relaxed and comfortable, and he could raise his arm much higher. He was still in pain and lacked some mobility, but he now had hope he could recover. His sub-sternal and abdominal pain upon pressing was diminished, so I used the same formula but halved the dose for another five packets. After taking the five packets, his abdominal presentation returned to normal. Later I treated him with acupuncture and herbs for another month and he made a complete recovery.

During the course of treatment, Pan De-fa told me certain things that had a deep impact on me and that I still remember now as if it were yesterday. He said that he had always been fairly healthy and this was the worst illness he'd been through in his whole life. He first sought treatment from western medicine, but after countless examinations and an eventual diagnosis of frozen shoulder, the treatment was entirely ineffective and he completely lost faith in western doctors. He then went to see a Chinese doctor. He found the Chinese doctor's diagnosis of qì and blood stagnation to be entirely reasonable, but after more than 100 packets of herbs, acupuncture, bloodletting and cupping, his condition only worsened and he once again lost hope. However, after taking my herbs, his faith in Chinese medicine was restored. He said that after a short exchange we had during the first visit, he felt a renewed sense of hope that his shoulder might recover. He had said that he didn't need abdominal palpation because his problem was in his shoulder, not his abdomen. I had told him that abdominal palpation had been used in Chinese medicine for millennia and in chronic disease, abdominal palpation was even more important than pulse-taking, as it was relatively objective and straightforward. When I palpated at his sub-sternum and lower left abdomen, he cried out in pain. When I told him these were clear diagnostic signs, it gave him renewed hope. He had been to many doctors over the last year, but not one had discovered that he had these painful areas in his abdomen.

During one visit, when he had already basically recovered, he asked me why other doctors didn't use abdominal palpation? He said he wanted to get his children to study Chinese medicine and asked me if I was willing to take on students. I said I was still learning myself and wasn't qualified to teach. He encouraged me and said I would certainly succeed. Five years later, I was already working at a city hospital. One day, while returning to the countryside, I heard someone call my name while I was passing over a bridge. When I looked down, I saw it was Pan De-fa rowing along the river in a canoe. He raised his right arm high up into the air and swung it all around while thanking me for healing him.

Abdominal palpation is an extremely important aspect of abdominal diagnosis. The first writings on abdominal palpation appear in the *Inner Canon* and the *Classic of Difficulties*. The diagnostic form later reached a high level of development and maturation in the *Treatise on Cold Damage*. Yumoto Kyūshin attached great importance to abdominal palpation or fukushin, in his *Imperial Han Medicine* he stated: "The abdomen is the source of life itself and is thus at the root of all disease. As such, abdominal palpation is an indispensable aspect of diagnosis." Keisetsu Ōtsuka, Dōmei Yakazu, and Takahide Sota have all echoed this view. The above patient had substernal glomus and pain upon pressing, signs consistent with a Xiao Xian Xiong Tang abdominal pattern. Additionally, the bind in the lower left abdomen and pain upon pressing with radiation of pain to the inguinal area is a classic Tao He Cheng Qi Tang abdominal pattern. Clearly, Tōdō Yoshimasu's statement that "one should not prescribe a formula if the abdominal pattern is unclear" are wise words indeed.

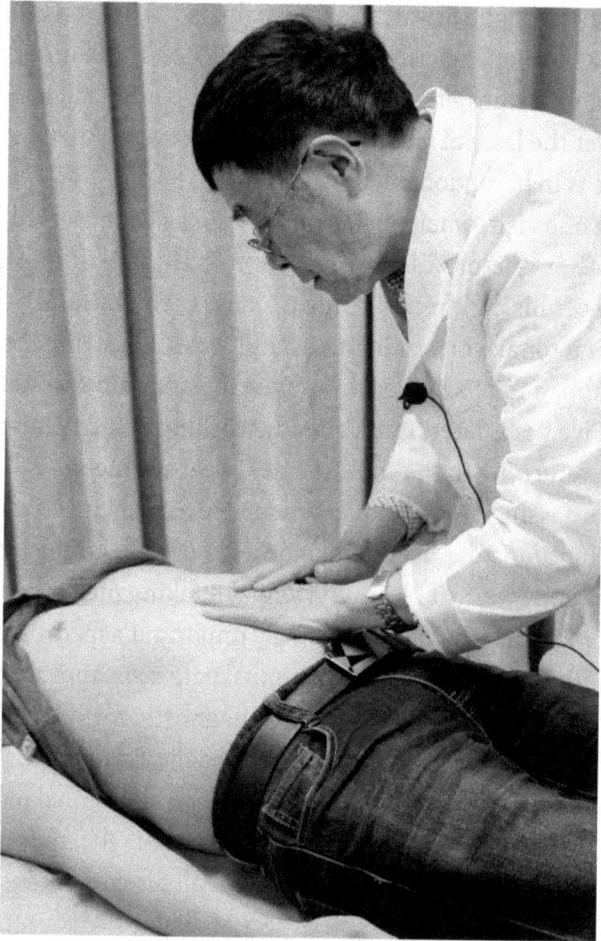

A Short Definition of Formula
Pattern Correspondence

Formula pattern correspondence refers to a correlation between the patient's symptom pattern and the established pattern for a formula or herb. The "patient's symptom pattern" refers to a diagnosis based on their clinical presentation—this diagnosis is guided by the unique, overarching classification scheme used in jīngfāng medicine. The "formula pattern" refers to the pattern which the formula in question is targeted to resolve. Together, they are like two sides of the same coin, and they will have corresponding symptoms, signs, pulses, tongue presentations, and abdominal presentations. For sake of clarity, the formula pattern is usually named using the formula used in the formula pattern in question. The formula pattern is a great treasure of our medicine, the bedrock of jīngfāng, and it has been proven through the trial-by-fire of clinical experimentation and practice in the long durée of Chinese medical history. As an example, take a patient with chronic gastritis that presents with stomach distention, eructation, chest oppression, and copious saliva. This presentation is consistent with a Xiang Su Yin formula pattern, so in such cases where correspondence is present, there is a high likelihood of efficacy.

Formula Pattern Correspondence is the Most Closely Aligned with Disease Patterns of Any Diagnostic System

The main reason why Chinese doctors are able to treat illness, be they jīngfāng practitioners or post-classical practitioners, is because they either knowingly or unknowingly make use of formula pattern diagnosis. That is to say, despite the fact that jīngfāng practitioners and post-classical practitioners might use different diagnostic methods, the fact that they are both capable of successfully treating illness suggests that they might arrive at the same destination by different paths.

Since ancient times, clinicians have always placed great importance on herbal formulas. From the Sui Dynasty *Categorized Formulas of the Four Seas* (四海類聚方), to the Jin Dynasty *Formulas for Emergency Use* (肘後備急方), to the Song Dynasty *Formulas from the Imperial Pharmacy* (太平惠民和劑局方), etc., the use of the word "formula" in the title of all these important tomes demonstrates the centrality of the formula in Chinese medicine.

Despite the fact that Li Dong-yuan used ideas from five element theory and viscera-bowel theory in his diagnosis, formula patterns and herb patterns were essential aspects of his actual practice. For instance, in his *Treatise on the Spleen and Stomach* he wrote this about using Wu Ling San: "(Wu Ling San) treats vexation thirst with excessive drinking of water or vomiting upon drinking water, sub-sternal splashing sound, stagnant dampness within and inhibited urine." As for Shao Yao Gan Cao Tang, he wrote: "It treats pain in the abdomen." Zhong Wan-chun (仲万春) noted: "In his *Changsha Formula Mnemonics* (長沙方歌訣), Chen Xiu-yuan (陳修園) clearly and directly argued that mastering the formulas of the *Treatise* should be the first step in training for practitioners of jīngfāng and Chinese clinical medicine in general. He wrote: 'The skill-set which new students and practitioners must master is to select the proper formulas for diseases based on the formula lineage of Yi Yin...'. Chen's categorization of patterns based on formula names indicates the orientation of his analysis." Indeed, Chen Xiu-yuan's orientation could not have been more clear—his was a clear early representation of the jīngfāng notions of formula pattern diagnosis and formula pattern correspondence.

If we imagine a disease pattern as the center of a circle which encompasses the entire nosology, the formula pattern occupies the layer closest to the center and all other diagnostic theories lie outside of it. Six-conformation diagnosis is closely nestled outside of formula pattern diagnosis, serving as a source of guidance, differentiation, comparison and verification. The more complicated a diagnostic and theoretical system becomes, the further it strays from the center and the less capable it will be of serving as an effective tool in clinic.

For instance, a jīngfāng practitioner will prescribe Xiao Xian Xiong Tang on the basis of the *Treatise* line, "In minor chest bind disease, (the site of illness) is below the sternum. If there is pain upon pressing there and a floating, slippery pulse, Xiao Xian Xiong Tang is indicated." As long as the pulse and abdominal presentation of the patient align with this pattern, the formula can be prescribed. Practitioners of the warm disease school take a similar approach. Despite stating in his *Treatise on Warm Heat* that Xiao Xian Xiong Tang is a bitter-acrid opening and downbearing method suitable for evil that has penetrated into the qì layer with phlegm-heating binding, Ye Tian-shi still noted that in clinical practice, diagnosis of the formula pattern must be based on the objective findings from the tongue. In a similar vein, Wang Meng-ying argued that the objective findings in the abdominal presentation should be the primary basis for diagnosis of a Xiao Xian Xiong Tang pattern. He wrote: "(When diagnosing), the chest and diaphragm must be palpated. If there is pain upon pressing or aversion to pressing, the tongue is red with a thick, yellow, greasy coating and the pulse slippery and rapid, first open and drain using Xiao Xian Xiong Tang." The *Treatise on Cold Damage* gives detailed descriptions of pulse and abdominal presentations in formula patterns, but more or less omits discussion of tongue presentations. From the above, we can see that warm disease practitioners also make use of formula pattern correspondence and helped flesh out formula patterns with important supplementary information regarding tongue presentation.

Reflections on Abdominal Patterns

Descriptions of abdominal presentations can be found throughout the *Treatise* and constitute an essential aspect of formula pattern diagnosis. Abdominal palpation is a relatively objective physical examination and is quite easy to learn. Strangely, this vital diagnostic method is rarely used in clinical practice in China. Indeed, I have yet to find a single abdominal pattern illustration in any book from the classical Chinese literature—why is this?

Classical Ruism emphasized the importance of governance while downplaying the role of science and technology. Those who engaged in scientific and technological research and development were mere "technicians" and had low societal status. In antiquity, it became fashionable for physicians to call themselves "Confucian doctors" and they took themselves to be a part of this "Ruist lineage". In Ruism, medicine was seen as a relatively lowly pursuit, but the belief was that physicians should still strive to uncover the mysteries of man in relation to the universe as well as the mechanistic basis of disease through the rubric of yīn-yáng theory. Any scientific discovery or breakthrough was relegated to the realm of "technology", a subject regarded as too vulgar for those of high Confucian cultivation. Confucianism promoted the idea that "the cultivated individual is not a "tool" or a specialist", "the cultivated individual works with his words, not with his hands" and "the cultivated individual disdains physicians, shamans, musicians and all others who engage in mere trades". These ideas limited intellectuals to a very narrow range of inquiry, discouraged any enthusiasm they may have had for scientific experimentation and cut them off from engaging with anyone that was doing real, tangible research and practice. Furthermore, centuries and perhaps even millennia of intellectuals were chastened by

the traumatic memory of the "burning of books and burying of scholars" during the Qin dynasty, such that they became subjugated by the
hierarchy of Confucian thought, dutifully offering prayers to the memo-
rial tablets of the "heaven, earth, sovereign, parents and teachers" while
losing all sense of intellectual experimentation and innovation. It is
primarily for this reason that we do not see any abdominal pattern illustrations in the classical Chinese medical literature.

With the introduction of the notion of "whimsical tinkering and
fanciful contriving" as a pejorative classification of scientific and technological inquiry in the Book of Documents (shàngshū, 書)
, it was inevitable that the juggernaut of scientific progress would be
adversely affected in China. Under the subtle influence of this societal
norm, intellectuals lost their enthusiasm for making sense of the natural
world surrounding them. With the atrophying of their critical faculties
and intellectual rigor, the Chinese lost their ability to think about the
world in novel ways and a period of conservative scholarship set in. In
truth, we lost the most important things of all: we lost our intellectual
frameworks, methods, logic, theory and our critical faculties, without which innovative thought becomes impossible. As we all know, the
Treatise on Cold Damage focuses on symptoms and signs and rarely discusses etiology of disease and pathomechanisms. Furthermore, the book
only lists formulas and rarely mentions anything about flavor, nature or
channel tropism. Thus, given the kind of intellectual climate that has
dominated China for the last two millennia, it's really no surprise that
the Treatise fell out of favor and that abdominal pattern illustrations
never surfaced.

With Tōdō Yoshimasu's proclamation that the "formulas of the
Treatise should be used, but not the theory", an emphasis on engagement
with Treatise formulas and a general spurning of theory became the norm
in the kampo school. This development was in complete opposition to the
Confucian call to pursue theory and downplay technology and science.
As such, the kampo school generally emphasized research into palpable,
objective forms of diagnosis, such as formula patterns and abdominal
patterns. They believed that the abdominal pattern was a special finding

that stood in close correspondence to its respective formula. Later on, *Extraordinary Views of Abdominal Patterns* (腹診奇覽) was published, a volume that featured illustrations for each abdominal pattern. These illustrations helped reinforce visual memory of the patterns and made the study of abdominal palpation that much easier and more convenient. In the "Fang Feng Tong Sheng San Abdominal Pattern" chapter of Yakazu Kaku's (矢数格) *Kampo Medicine of Ikkandō* (漢方一貫堂醫學), Kaku writes: "Fang Feng Tong Sheng San is not a formula of the the jīngfāng canon and was originally understood as a formula for resolving the exterior and interior in exterior heat disease. The contemporary *kampo* practitioner Mori Dōhaku (森道伯) found an innovative new use for this formula. He said that this was the best formula for improving the constitution of those with an organ toxicity constitution[23]." In complex, chronic patients that present with the Fang Feng Tong Sheng San abdominal pattern, a strong build and a propensity to constipation, this formula can be quite effective. This formula's abdominal pattern features a strong, full abdomen with distention and binding centered around the navel. The illustration for the pattern vividly portrays the peri-umbilical fullness, distention and binding, displaying concentric rings fanning out from the navel. These abdominal pattern illustrations displayed alongside written descriptions leave a deeper impact on the student and provide a stronger visual representation of the pattern in question. The contemporary *kampo* physician Mori Dōhaku enumerated three primary constitutions: Blood stagnation constitution, organ toxicity constitution and scrofulous constitution[24]. This broad classification allowed physicians to make a general diagnosis of patients as soon as they walked into the clinic. By studying his work, one gains a clear picture of the causal relationship between constitution and disease. A patient with Mori's organ toxicity constitution will have a strong build and will often be quite healthy in their youth and middle age, but they have high mortality rates as seniors due to their propensity to develop hypertension, coronary artery disease,

---

[23] A constitution marked by a propensity to accumulate food toxicity, water toxicity, and syphilis.

[24] A constitution characterized by a tendency towards exudation into the skin and mucous membranes. Mori often used Chai Hu Qing Gan Tang to treat this constitution.

diabetes, kidney atrophy etc. The Japanese *kampo* school developed abdominal diagnosis much later than the *Classic of Difficulties* and only began being incorporating it into clinical practice in the early years of the Edo period. Practitioners such as Tōdō Yoshimasu and Inaba Bunrei played pivotal roles in the advancement of this new diagnostic practice.

Fang Feng Tong Sheng San has a wide range of application in clinic. For patients with hyperlipidemia or hypertension that possess the Fang Feng Tong Sheng San abdominal pattern, long-term usage of Fang Feng Tong Sheng San pills is very effective. Oddly, the manufacturer that makes the Fang Feng Tong Sheng San pills states that they are contraindicated in hypertension!

Dr. Feng Shi-lun (馮世綸) made the following comment regarding abdominal diagnosis: "The idea of abdominal patterns originates from the *Treatise on Cold Damage*. Abdominal diagnosis is a very important aspect of clinical practice. The Japanese and Koreans have done some research on this topic and created something called "abdomen-based treatment". As the name would suggest, in "abdomen-based treatment", the treatment strategy is formulated based upon the abdominal pattern diagnosed. For instance, if they diagnose a Da Huang Fu Zi Xi Xin Tang abdominal pattern, that is the formula they will use. This approach is overly dependent on abdominal diagnosis. In reality, the *Treatise* details several forms of formula pattern correspondence, so we shouldn't rely solely on abdominal diagnosis, but should consider all symptoms and signs together. There are many abdominal patterns detailed in the *Treatise* and they are all quite important. What does Zhong-jing mean by "stomach domain repletion". There are actually several possible formula patterns grouped under "stomach domain repletion". Da Cheng Qi Tang for instance, must present with a particular abdominal pattern, but Zhi Zi Chi Tang, which also falls under "stomach domain repletion", does not have a abdominal pattern. Da Chai Hu Tang's "urgency below the heart" is a kind of abdominal pattern—how would you ascertain a diagnosis in this case without abdominal palpation. "Urgency below the heart" refers both to the patient's subjective experience and the avoidance of the patient upon palpating that area."

A Commentary on Line 106 of the *Treatise*

Line 106 states: "When tàiyáng disease fails to resolve, heat binds in the urinary bladder, and the patient has symptoms similar to mania, if they spontaneously bleed below, the illness will resolve. If the external condition has not resolved, the internal condition should not be attacked. The external condition should first be resolved. If the external condition resolves but there is still binding urgency in the lower lateral abdomen, an attacking method can be used. Tao He Cheng Qi Tang can be used."

At first glance, this line seems to resemble a shàoyáng yángmíng dragover disease. The "external" in the "if the external condition has not resolved" above requires some close analysis.

In the Japanese *kampo* tradition, they have developed a methodology for decoding classical Chinese that often unravels the hidden meaning buried deep within the text. The key to this passage is the use of the word "external" (外) as opposed to "exterior" (表). "External" refers to tàiyáng and shàoyáng. Paired with "external" is "internal", which here refers to the Tao He Cheng Qi Tang pattern. The use of the word "external", is a roundabout way of telling us there is a Xiao Chai Hu Tang pattern. The external and internal conditions combine to constitute a shàoyáng yángmíng dragover disease. This line is describing how heat from tàiyáng disease binds with blood and becomes a blood stagnation pattern. If there is also concurrently an external condition, the external condition should first be resolved before attacking the stagnant blood. There are cases in which Gui Zhi Tang is employed to treat "external" conditions, but from the fact that this line makes specific use of the word "external" and avoids "exterior", it would seem more likely that this is referring to a Xiao Chai Hu Tang pattern.

Line 106 is like a polygonal prism; it is not so easy to view it clearly. I have conducted deeper analysis of the line, but even then, it is ultimately just my opinion, and one can just take it for what it's worth. That being said, there is value in delving deeper into this line—by studying it, one can draw closer to Zhong-jing's original thought process, which will be helpful in clinic. "If the external condition hasn't resolved" is Zhong-jing's way of signaling that there is still an internal condition. Wang Ang (汪昂) wrote: "In Zhong-jing's writings, he always signaled that there was an internal condition by saying "if the exterior has not resolved", but "if the external condition has not resolved" also hints at the existence of an internal condition." I would argue that "if the external condition has not resolved" suggests that there is a tàiyáng-shàoyáng combination disease. Combined with the interior condition, the entire diagnosis then becomes tàiyáng-shàoyáng combination disease plus yángmíng Tao He Cheng Qi Tang dragover disease.

The Indispensability of Gui Zhi in the *Treatise*

In the original Gui Zhi Tang dosage, Gui Zhi is dosed at 3 liang (90g), the equivalent of about 1.5 liang (45g) by modern measurements. In my book, *A Life Devoted to Chinese Medicine* (中醫人生), I recounted the story of a famous Wenzhou physician named Jin Shen-zhi who was disgraced when a patient of his died after he accidentally prescribed her Six qian (18g) of Gui Zhi. Six qian (錢) is just 2/5 of 1.5 liang. Even the very lowest dose conversion method puts Gui Zhi at 3 qián, which 6 qián is only double the dose of. This is well within the safety standards of Chinese herbal pharmacology. Indeed, Gui Zhi has been used in cooking for it's fragrant spice and positive effects on the stomach — it's completely non-toxic, so it would be an absolute joke to argue that Gui Zhi can be lethal.

The idea that Gui Zhi can cause iatrogenic effects likely derives from a line in the *Treatise* which states: "In patients with yáng repletion, Gui Zhi can cause instant death." Additionally, in the tàiyáng chapter of the *Treatise*, Zhong-jing writes: "One should not give Gui Zhi Tang to drinkers and alcoholics. They will vomit upon taking Gui Zhi Tang because drinkers are averse to sweet things. For those that vomit upon taking Gui Zhi Tang, they will certainly vomit thick blood later on." This is to say, in patients with replete yáng heat conditions, Gui Zhi Tang can have adverse effects.

The first formula in the *Treatise* is Gui Zhi Tang, just as the first formula in the *Essential Prescriptions of the Golden Cabinet* is Gua Lou Gui Zhi Tang. Zhong-jing invested a deep hidden meaning into the structure of his works, but later commentators haven't paid this much attention or have passed over it due to familiarity. Gui Zhi has a privileged status in the *Treatise*, appearing in 43 of the 112 formulas listed. It is truly an indispensable herb in the jīngfāng canon. Removing Gui Zhi from the *Treatise*

292 THE JINGFANG CASE STUDIES AND MEDICAL TREATISES

would be like removing its backbone or central pillar, which is why the story of Jin Shen-zhi is so regrettable.[25] In his *Collected Medical Treatises of Dr. Lu*, Lu Yuan-lei stated: "I have used Gui Zhi thousands of times and never once seen a case of adverse reactions, much less has anyone died as a result of taking it. Physicians needn't worry at all about the safety of this herb." In the book, he recounts how as a young student he developed a bad cough after getting a cold and went to his acupuncture teacher seeking treatment. The teacher diagnosed it as a "urinary bladder cough" and prescribed Gui Zhi Tang plus 9g of Bei Mu and 9g of Xing Ren. To his amazement, after just two doses, the cough completely resolved.

Ge Gen Tang, which features Ma Huang in combination with Gui Zhi, is the first-choice formula for exterior contraction with heat effusion. In the *Divine Farmer's Materia Medica* and the *Treatise*, Ma Huang, Gui Zhi and other warm, acrid herbs are used to resolve the exterior and abate heat. The famous Daoist philosopher and Southern dynasty physician Tao Hong-jing (陶弘景) emphatically stated: "Ma Huang is the first-choice herb for treating cold damage and resolving the flesh." This statement is clearly quoted in Li Shi-zhen's Ben Cao Gang Mu (Compendium of Materia Medica), and yet most versions of the modern *Chinese Internal Medicine* textbooks seem to omit formulas containing these two herbs.

As a remedy to the strange phenomenon in society whereby physicians and laypeople seemed to have an irrational fear of Gui Zhi, Lu Yuan-lei heavily promoted the study of Yoshimasu's *Herbal Patterns* (藥徵), because this book interpreted the nature of herbs based upon their usage in the *Treatise* and the *Essential Prescriptions of the Golden Cabinet*. For instance, regarding Gui Zhi's nature, Yoshimasu wrote: "Gui Zhi is primarily indicated for the treatment of upward surging and

---

[25] Jin Shen-zhi was a famous Qing dynasty doctor. As the story goes, one day he was called to treat the wife of an aristocrat who had come down with a cold. He prescribed her Gui Zhi Tang, but used a very small dose (1.5g) because he knew that patient had a very weak constitution. The next day, however, the woman died after taking the medication. When he was summoned before a local magistrate to explain what had happened, he said that it was nearly impossible that the formula could have contributed to her death and requested to examine the herbs used in the decoction. As it turned out, the pharmacy had misread the dosage of Gui Zhi as 15g instead of 1.5g and this accounted for the adverse reaction. (Dr. Lou says it was 18g in his book, but the translator can only find records of using 15g.)

counterflow." To the average Chinese physician, this might seem like an absurd statement, but upon closer examination of the *Treatise* and the *Essential Prescriptions*, one finds that Zhong-jing actually made abundant use of Gui Zhi in this capacity. For instance, the *Treatise* states: "In tàiyáng disease, if after purging, qì surges upwards, Gui Zhi Tang can be used. If there is no upward surging, Gui Zhi Tang should not be used." Clearly, upward surging is a primary indicator for the use of Gui Zhi. The *Treatise* also states: "In running piglet disease, when qì surges upwards from the lower abdomen, Gui Zhi Jia Gui Tang can be used." This line also appears in the *Essential Prescriptions*.

Gui Zhi Tang is Not Just an Exterior Resolving Formula

A formula's action and its clinical usage are separate but related concepts, however modern formulary textbooks do a bad job at articulating this fact. For instance, Gui Zhi Tang's primary action is to harmonize construction and defense and supplement qì and blood, so its strengthening and supplementing effects are exploited in patients with exterior vacuity and an absence of sweating to resolve the flesh and promote sweating. Likewise, in patients with exterior vacuity and spontaneous sweating, its strengthening and supplementing effect is deployed to constrain sweating and secure the exterior.

Why did Zhong-jing place Gui Zhi Tang, a formula with a harmonizing and supplementing action, as the first formula for treating exterior contraction in tàiyáng disease?

This is what sets the Treatise apart from other texts. It would stand to reason that Ma Huang Tang should be the first formula discussed in a chapter about exterior contraction, because it represents the standard way of treating exterior contraction with acrid, dispersing herbs that promote sweating and resolve the exterior. Gui Zhi Tang, in turn, should be placed after Ma Huang Tang, as it is a non-standard approach to exterior contraction involving supplementing and harmonizing construction and defense. Zhong-jing believed that the treatment of disease follows certain predictable patterns, but diseases themselves often also develop in unpredictable ways. As such, clinical physicians must be capable of following protocols, but also adapting to circumstances and unpredictable dynamics of disease. This latter quality is often even more important than the former.

Gui Zhi Tang is the Centerpiece of Zhong-jing's Formula Repertoire

Gui Zhi Tang is the first formula listed in the *Treatise* and modifications of Gui Zhi Tang account for over 20 formulas in that tome. In the Edo Period Koho lineage leader Nagoya Gen-I's (名古屋玄醫) *Medical Formula Protocols* (醫方規矩), most of the formulas he lists are modifications of Gui Zhi Tang. Nagoya Gen-I's approach strongly embodied the true meaning and clinical value of Ke Qin's (柯琴) assertion that "Gui Zhi Tang is the centerpiece of Zhong-jing's Formula Repertoire".

Gui Zhi Tang is not only a tàiyáng disease formula pattern, it also has internal connections to the primary formula patterns of all six conformations. This connection is typically manifested via combination formulas with primary formula patterns of the six conformations. I will review these combinations in detail below.

1. The Gui Zhi Tang formula pattern is connected to the tàiyáng disease Ma Huang Tang formula pattern via the Gui Zhi Ma Huang Ge Ban Tang formula pattern.

2. The Gui Zhi Tang formula pattern is connected to the yángmíng replete bowel disease Cheng Qi Tang patterns via the Gui Zhi Jia Da Huang Tang formula pattern.

3. The Gui Zhi Tang formula pattern is connected to the yángmíng qì phase Bai Hu Tang pattern via the Gui Zhi Er Yue Bi Yi Tang formula pattern.

4. The Gui Zhi Tang formula pattern is connected to the shàoyáng disease Xiao Chai Hu Tang formula pattern via the Chai Hu Gui Zhi Tang formula pattern.

5. The Gui Zhi Tang formula pattern is connected to the shàoyáng disease Huang Qin Tang formula pattern via the Shao Yao Gan Cao Tang formula pattern.

6. The Gui Zhi Tang formula pattern is connected to the tàiyáng disease Xiao Jian Zhong Tang formula pattern via the Gui Zhi Jia Shao Yao Tang formula pattern.

7. The Gui Zhi Tang formula pattern is connected to the Tàiyīn disease Li Zhong Tang pattern via the Gui Zhi Ren Shen Tang formula pattern.

8. The Gui Zhi Tang formula pattern is connected to the shàoyīn disease Si Ni Tang formula pattern via the Gui Zhi Jia Fu Zi Tang formula pattern.

9. The Gui Zhi Tang formula pattern is connected to the shàoyīn disease Zhen Wu Tang formula pattern via the Shao Yao Gan Cao Jia Fu Zi Tang formula pattern.

10. The Gui Zhi Tang formula pattern is connected to the Juéyīn disease Wu Mei Wan formula pattern via the Chai Hu Gui Zhi Gan Jiang Tang formula pattern.

Gui Zhi Tang is also the base formula whose modifications treat all manner of qì, blood and water derangements.

1. Gui Zhi Jia Gui Tang treats "qì surging upwards into the chest".

2. Gui Zhi Tang qu Shao Yao treats "rapid pulse and full chest" due to obstruction of qì in the chest.

3. Gui Tang qu Gui Jia Fu Ling Bai Zhu treats congestion of water qì leading to "sub-sternal fullness and slight pain with inhibited urine".

4. Fu Ling Gui Zhi Gan Cao Da Zao Tang treats "sub-umbilical palpitations" due to water qì overflowing upwards.

5. Fu Ling Gui Zhi Bai Zhu Gan Cao Tang treats "sub-sternal counterflow and fullness, qì surging upwards to the chest and dizziness upon standing" due to counterflow of water qì.

6. Wu Ling San can be traced back to Gui Zhi Tang via Fu Ling Gui Zhi Bai Zhu Gan Cao Tang. Wu Ling San treats "vomiting upon drinking water" due to lack of transformation of water qì and subsequent counterflow.

7. Zhen Wu Tang can be traced back to Gui Zhi Tang via Shao Yao Gan Cao Fu Zi Tang. Zhen Wu Tang treats "sub-sternal palpitations, dizziness, spasms and poor balance with likelihood of falling" due to yáng deficiency and water overflow.

8. Tao He Cheng Qi Tang can be seen as a distant modification of Gui Zhi Tang. This formula treats heat-stagnation binding leading to "urgent binding in the lower lateral abdomen".

Explaining Gui Zhi Tang from Four Different Perspectives

EXPLAINING GUI ZHI TANG FROM THE PERSPECTIVE OF ITS CONSTITUENT HERBS

Gui Zhi Tang is made up of five herbs; upon deeper analysis, this Zhongjing formula can be divided into three sub-units, each with its own indications.

Gui Zhi Gan Cao sub-unit. Indications: Palpitations, sweating, headache.

Shao Yao Gan Cao sub-unit. Indications: Abdominal pain, leg pain, headache.

Sheng Jiang Da Zao sub-unit. Indications: In the formative period of formula creation, ancient peoples found that this sub-unit stimulates the appetite and protects the GI tract, so it was often combined with all other sub-units for this purpose. Later on, they found that this sub-unit would diminish the effect of certain formulas, so it was removed. This is why the Sheng Jiang Da Zao sub-unit can be found in nearly half of all Treatise formulas.

If a patient presented with palpitations, sweating, headache, and abdominal pain, their symptom presentation would be consistent with the indications from two of the sub-units, so Gui Zhi, Shao Yao, and Gan Cao would be prescribed. The effect of this combination was amplified by adding Sheng Jiang and Da Zao to strengthen and protect stomach qì. Through a process of repeated clinical experimentation, this combination was found to be reliably effective and became an established multi-sub-unit formula.

Later on, this multi-sub-unit formula was gradually tried out in other scenarios. For instance, it was later found that it was also effective in treating patients with headache, sweating, heat effusion, aversion to cold, and aversion to wind. After a long process of clinical evaluation, it was found to be reliably effective in this scenario. Thus, "heat effusion, aversion to cold, and aversion to wind" were added to the multi-sub-unit formula's indications.

Through this process of iterative expansion of indications and experimentation with different sub-units, Gui Zhi Tang's herbal components and formula pattern were gradually established over the long durée of history.

Deconstructing Gui Zhi Tang into its constituent sub-units and understanding the formula patterns of each sub-unit is extremely beneficial for a deeper knowledge of the formula.

Gui Zhi Tang's Indications

Gui Zhi Tang's indications can be classified into five major sub-categories: 1.) Weak constitution, thin build, a history of illness as a child including prolonged or high fevers, and swollen lymph nodes. 2.) Aversion to wind, aversion to cold and sweating. 3.) Tightness in the rectus abdominis. 4.) In acute and infectious disease, apart from aversion to cold and sweating, there should also be heat effusion. 5.) In chronic disease, heat effusion need not be present.

Two Blind Spots in the Clinical Use of Gui Zhi Tang

1. Many people don't dare use Gui Zhi Tang in external contraction with heat effusion due to a mischaracterization of external contraction disease. In modern times, external contraction is often divided into externally contracted wind-heat and externally contracted wind-cold.

Externally contracted wind-cold is said to be marked by a floating and tight or moderate pulse, whereas externally contracted wind-heat will have a rapid pulse.

However, in clinical reality, all patients with external contraction may present with a rapid pulse if their fever is sufficiently high. This is to say that externally contracted wind-cold may also present with a rapid pulse, on top of a floating and tight pulse. The mechanical use of cool, acrid formulas like Yin Qiao San and Sang Ju Yin whenever a rapid pulse presents has led to the diminished used of Ma Huang Tang, Ge Gen Tang, and Da Qing Long Tang. As such, Gui Zhi Tang stopped being used in externally contracted febrile disease.

2. Very few people use Gui Zhi Tang to treat miscellaneous conditions. The reason for this is that miscellaneous conditions (such as dermatological diseases, joint pain, or autonomic disorders) that present with spontaneous sweating and headache often won't be accompanied by symptoms associated with external contraction, and most textbooks say that Gui Zhi Tang can only be used in external conditions. As such, people are afraid to use it. In actuality, Gui Zhi Tang was first used for miscellaneous diseases and only later was adopted for use in externally contracted febrile disease. Feng Shi-lun also holds this view. In his article "Experience in Treating Impediment Disease"[26] he wrote: "Through their experience in treating impediment disease pain, the ancients developed a systematic understanding of the nature of disease. They termed exterior replete heat patterns tàiyáng disease, exterior vacuity cold patterns as shàoyīn disease and, in this way, also classified interior and half interior half exterior patterns according to a yīn-yáng classification scheme. This is the origin of the six-conformation system.

Simply put, some physicians are under the misconception that Gui Zhi Tang cannot be used in cases of heat effusion with a rapid pulse, while others fail to grasp the principal symptoms in the Gui Zhi Tang formula pattern. Gui Zhi Tang can be used in external contraction with

---

[26] Published in *100 Great Clinicians of China—Hu Xi-shu*, 2001 (中国百名临床家丛书 ——胡希恕).

heat effusion, but in miscellaneous diseases the Gui Zhi Tang formula pattern need not include heat effusion. However, in most modern textbooks, heat effusion is listed as an integral symptom in the Gui Zhi Tang formula pattern. As a result, many people fail to prescribe Gui Zhi Tang in miscellaneous diseases that call for this formula because they are limited by this notion that the Gui Zhi Tang formula pattern includes heat effusion. In external contraction with heat effusion Gui Zhi Tang can be used, but in miscellaneous diseases that do not present with heat effusion, Gui Zhi Tang can also be used. This is a very important point—if one fails to grasp this concept, they will have a hard time using Gui Zhi Tang effectively.

4. Regarding the use of Gui Zhi Tang in Patients with and without Spontaneous Sweating

Can Gui Zhi Tang be used in a patient with a weak constitution, aversion to wind, aversion to cold, and an absence of spontaneous sweating? Much to the surprise of many, the answer is yes!

In a patient with aversion to cold, aversion to wind, a weak constitution, and an absence of sweating, one can use pulse to determine whether it is appropriate to use Gui Zhi Tang. If the pulse is floating and moderate, and has a slack quality to it, Gui Zhi Tang can be used.

If the patient has a strong constitution, the pulse is floating and tight, and there is no sweating, Ma Huang Tang should be used instead of Gui Zhi Tang.

In the majority of cases, the Gui Zhi Tang pattern presents with sweating, but there are always exceptions to the rule. In some situations, if the patient has a relatively weak constitution and an absence of sweating, but they have aversion to wind and cold and a slack, moderate pulse, Gui Zhi Tang can still be used.

Indeed, some Gui Zhi Tang lines do not include pulse. For instance, Line 13 in the Song dynasty version of the Treatise does not include pulse, it just lists the standard symptoms of aversion to cold, aversion to wind, headache, and spontaneous sweating. If those standard symptoms present, one can use Gui Zhi Tang. However, if the person has aversion to wind and cold, headache, and no sweating, the pulse should be used to perform differential diagnosis. If the pulse is tight and the person has a stronger constitution, use Ma Huang Tang. If the pulse is slack and the constitution is relatively weak, then even if the patient is not sweating, Ma Huang Tang shouldn't be used.

In this sense, pulse can be a reflection of a patient's constitution. Gui Zhi Tang can be used in patients with spontaneous sweating and in patients with an absence of sweating.

Ma Huang Fu Zi Xi Xin Tang is The First Choice for Febrile Exterior Contraction in Weak Constitutions

During the Cultural Revolution, my 3-year-old nephew once ran a fever that lasted for over two weeks. My brother-in-law was locally known as a famous pediatrician and he treated his son with various antibiotics, but the fever failed to abate. I happened to visit my sister while my nephew had this fever, and my sister asked me to prescribe something for him because my brother-in-law had gone out of town. Upon questioning, I learned that my nephew had only just recovered from measles when he developed this cold. His face was extremely palid, he seemed fatigued and dejected, and his temperature was 38.3°C. His symptom presentation seemed to align with a Ma Huang Fu Zi Xi Xin Tang pattern. My brother-in-law's uncle thought that the child should continue using penicillin because he had a high white blood cell count and my brother-in-law's father, who had some understanding of Chinese medicine, said that using a warming formula like Ma Huang Fu Zi Xi Xin Tang in heat effusion, which he perceived to be a "warm condition", would be extremely dangerous. However, I was very confident in my diagnosis and insisted on prescribing Ma Huang Fu Zi Xi Xin Tang, despite the dissenting opinions of my relatives. On the following day, my nephew seemed more energetic, his fever abated, and his white blood cell count also decreased. I followed up with Xiao Jian Zhong Tang for a week, after which his white blood cell count returned to normal, and he made a complete recovery.

The shàoyīn disease Ma Huang Fu Zi Xi Xin Tang formula pattern, which is also called an exterior yīn pattern, is extremely common in clinic. In my extensive experience with using this formula, I have found there is really no substitute for it when treating external febrile disease in weak constitutions. In the south of China, where I live, many doctors are afraid of using warm herbs because they believe they're not suited to our warm, damp climate, but this is an unsubstantiated extrapolation. In the *kampo* tradition, Ma Huang Fu Zi Xi Xin tang is believed to be the first-choice formula for febrile exterior contraction in children or elderly people with weak constitutions. Clearly, it is quite important to learn from the research and experimentation of the *kampo* tradition.

Treatment of "Water Toxicity" with Ling Gui Zhu Gan Tang.

Ling Gui Zhu Gan Tang is an extremely important formula. I have treated several cases of orthostatic vertigo, or as the *Treatise* states, "vertigo upon rising", using this formula. In general, these patients tend to also have anemia and orthostatic hypotension which I often address with combinations of other formulas. Using a *kampo* style of analysis, these patients all had what they call "water toxicity"; they would have sub-sternal palpitations, splash sound upon tapping on the stomach, inhibited urine, and a wet, pale, engorged and scalloped tongue. In this formula, Fu Ling is the principal herb and can be dosed to 30g or above. Water toxicity patients have a primary dysfunction of water metabolism and secondary dysfunction of qì transformation. This is why Fu Ling has the highest dose, while Gui Zhi has a slightly lower dose. If the patient presents with Gui Zhi's herbal pattern, namely "sub-sternal fullness and counterflow with qì upsurging to the chest", Gui Zhi's dosage can be increased.

CASE STUDY EXAMPLE

MS. LI, 35 YEARS

HISTORY: The patient has suffered from dizziness for six years with exacerbation of the symptom in the last 2 months which has forced her to take sick leave. She was diagnosed with anemia (hemoglobin: 9.3g/l) by western medicine and treatment has been unsatisfactory. Chinese medical physicians also previously prescribed qì and blood supplementing herbs with little effect. Her parents, husband and two children are all in good health.

CURRENT: The patient is slightly overweight, has a ghostly pallid complexion and slight edema in the face. She complains of heaviness in the head, vertigo, palpitations, panicky feeling in the chest, shortness of breath, light sleep, and cold hands and feet. Her rectus abdominis was quite tight and her tongue was pale with a glossy coating. Her pulse was thin and soft.

DIAGNOSIS: Water toxicity leading to blood vacuity.

I informed her that the treatment would mainly focus on draining water toxicity, while also supplementing blood and that treatment might take as long as 6 months to completely resolve the condition.

I prescribed Lian Zhu Yin (Ling Gui Zhu Gan Tang plus Si Wu Tang).

After one month, her complexion improved. After three months, she was able to return to work, her symptoms all resolved, and her hemoglobin rose to 10.2g/L. After another month of herbs, she reported being in good health and her period volume increased.

Li Dong-yuan Was a Good Student
of Zhang Zhong-jing

What is Li Dong-yuan's most important formula? It has to be Bu Zhong Yi Qi Tang.

Much like Zhang Zhong-jing's Gui Zhi Tang, Li Dong-yuan's Bu Zhong Yi Qi Tang encapsulates the very essence of Li Dong-yuan's approach to medicine. Like Gui Zhi Tang, Bu Zhong Yi Qi Tang's main action is harmonizing construction and defense and supplementing middle qì, but also similar to Gui Zhi Tang, Bu Zhong Yi Qi Tang can resolve the exterior and abate heat in patients with weak constitutions that contract external febrile disease. This is why I believe Li Dong-yuan was a good student of Zhang Zhong-jing. The only book that Li produced in his lifetime, *Treatise on Differential Diagnosis of Internal and External Damage* (內外傷辨惑論), was not only a book about spleen and stomach pathophysiology, it also addressed the treatment of external febrile disease and pandemic disease. As Zhang Jing-yue (張景岳) stated: "In patients with damage to the spleen due to taxation and middle qì vacuity who develop febrile exterior contraction, Bu Zhong Yi Qi Tang is indicated." While reading *Treatise on Differential Diagnosis of Internal and External Damage*, I noticed that Li Dong-yuan also mimics Zhong-jing's literary style. Lines like "If there is mutual contention of wind and damp and pain throughout the body, Chu Feng Shi Qiang Huo Tang is indicated" and "If there is back and shoulder pain, spontaneous sweating, and scant and frequent urination, this is wind-heat overwhelming the lung. In cases where lung qì is severely congested, draining wind-heat will resolve the condition. Tong Qi Fang Feng Tang is indicated" are all redolent of Zhong-jing's literary style.

Be Weary of Fu Zi and Wu Tou Poisoning

Kampo practitioners have a strong respect for the clinical efficacy of Wu Tou and Fu Zi. Dōmei Yakazu's PhD thesis involved research into Fu Zi. He argued that Fu Zi is the best cardiotonic medicine in the world. However, practitioners in the *kampo* school are very careful about how they use Fu Zi because the revered 19th-20th century herbalist Mitsutaro Shirai died from poisoning associated with Fu Zi.

Yakazu found Wu Tou and Fu Zi contain six kinds of aconitine alkaloids. The first four contain toxic compounds, while the last two contain curative compounds. The first four compounds can be denatured at high temperatures, while the last two are preserved at high temperatures. After a prolonged process of experimentation, the Osaka University professor Shintaro Takahashi (高橋真太郎) developed a method for preparing "non-toxic Fu Zi". This prepared Fu Zi has already been approved for use and is available on the mass market in Kosei province in Japan. The method for preparing the non-toxic Fu Zi is quite simple: Fu Zi is placed in a pressure cooker and heated at 120°C for 2 hours.

Zhong-jing's method for preparing Wu Tou: In Wu Tou Gui Zhi Tang, 21g of Wu Tou are immersed in 90g of honey for one hour. After one hour, the Wu Tou honey immersion is cooked in a pot until the honey is on the verge of drying completely. The remaining decoction is then added to a pot of water with the components of Gui Zhi Tang and decocted for 2 hours. As for consumption of Wu Tou, Zhong-jing emphasizes starting at a low dose and slowly increasing the dose to avoid poisoning. The principal symptoms of the Wu Tou Gui Zhi Tang pattern are back pain and cold numbness in the four limbs. This correlates well with the *Essential Prescriptions* description of the Wu Tou Gui Zhi Tang pattern: "Abdominal pain, coldness and numbness in the hands and feet and body pain". In his *Golden Cabinet Formula Mnemonics* (金匱方歌括), Chen Xiu-yuan writes: "For abdominal pain, body pain and numbness of the limbs, acupuncture, moxibustion and other herbal treatments will not do. Decoct Gui Zhi Tang normally and combine it with Wu Tou that has been cooked in honey."

Reading "On My Studies" from
The Medical Treatises of Yue Mei-zhong

Physicians should have a foundation in a systematic understanding of medical theory and practice, but they should not become biased towards one way or aspect of practice. In "On My Studies" from Yue Mei-zhong's *The Medical Treatises of Yue Mei-zhong* (岳美中醫话集), Yue states: "In the jīngfāng tradition, there is a particular emphasis on warming and supplementing. If the diagnosis is just slightly off, the prescription can often have a highly deleterious effect on the condition of the patient. If one adopts ideological biases in their practice of medicine, they will develop an inaccurate understanding of medical truths. As the saying goes: 'Just one mote of dust in the eye can throw off one's grasp of the four cardinal directions.' A bias can prevent a physician from delivering effective care." These are wise words. The Fire Spirit School is an example of this kind of ideological predisposition to one aspect of disease. It represents an over-correction and is certainly not a mainstream approach in Chinese medicine. The following is an excerpt from "On My Studies":

I began studying medicine when none of the doctors I saw could cure a chronic pulmonological disease I developed that left me coughing up blood and short of breath. It was a difficult process full of setbacks and continual progressions and reversals in my ideological development. My development as a physician progressed through three major stages: In the first stage, I was mainly reading Zhang Xi-chun's (張錫純) *On Medicine: Chinese at Heart and Western as Reference* (醫學衷中參西錄) and mostly prescribed post-classical formulas. After practicing for a while, I found this approach limiting, and so I began studying warm disease through the works of Wu Ju-tong (吳鞠通) and Wang Meng-ying (王孟英), however I found their approach to be too complicated and their formulas too weak. I began to wonder how Chinese medicine, which had been developing for nearly 4,000 years, could produce such middling results. Was it the medicine itself, or had I yet to find the right approach? In the midst of my searching, I went back to reading the *Treatise* and the *Essential Prescriptions* and noted how they diagnosed patterns without resort to theory, prescribed formulas without discussing the nature of the herbs used and seemed to base treatment on objective findings. The direct, empirical nature of this approach seemed more scientific and proved to be quite useful in clinic. Later on, I went on to study the *Essential Formulas Worth a Thousand in Gold* and *Essential Secrets from the External Official Library* and found that they seemed to pick up right where Zhong Jing left off—they were practical and empirical volumes that also translated to excellent clinical results. From 1934 to 1949, I only used classical formulas and often used them to effectively treat difficult diseases. I became increasingly convinced that the true greatness of Chinese medicine lay in the works of the pre-Song period. During that time period, I obsessively poured over medical works from the Han to Tang dynasties and benefited greatly from my study. This was the first period.

Gradually, in the course of my studies, I began to find that using only classical formulas just wasn't enough. Firstly, as I began to see a greater diversity of illnesses, I realized that I just didn't have enough methods and approaches in my arsenal to take on every disease that came my way. Secondly, in the jīngfāng tradition, there is a particular emphasis on warming and supplementing. If the diagnosis is just slightly off, the prescription can often have a highly deleterious effect on the condition of the patient. If one adopts ideological biases in their practice of medicine, they will develop an inaccurate understanding of medical truths. As the saying goes: 'Just one mote of dust in the eye can throw off one's grasp of the four cardinal directions.' A bias can prevent a physician from delivering effective care." From the end of the 40s to the beginning of the 50s, I gained a new understanding through a process of study, discussion with colleagues and clinical practice. I found that *Treatise* formulas can be overly strong, whereas warm disease formulas can be overly weak.

Strong formulas can cause severe side effects, while weak formulas fail to achieve results at all. I knew I had to garner a deeper understanding of classical formulas and take a practical approach to the use of post-classical formulas. Gaining a deeper understanding would help simplify the complexity, while taking a practical approach would lead to better results in difficult cases. During that period of study, I came to the following conclusion: Zhong-jing's jīngfāng should be used to treat difficult and severe cases. Li Dong-yuan's formula repertoire is best suited for treating gastrointestinal disease, while Ye Tian-shi's formulas could be referenced in the treatment of warm disease and less severe disease. In sum, the only way to avoid bias and address disease accurately and effectively, was to select formulas based on the person, the pattern, the season and the geographical location. This was my second period of study.

From 1954 onward, I began studying dialectical materialism and applied this knowledge to my previous medical experience and ideology to gain yet a new perspective. I found that insisting on using old formulas to treat modern people was often impractical, regardless of how much I strove to blend ancient and contemporary, eastern and western approaches. However, abandoning classical medicine would also leave me without a system to operate within. To avoid this dilemma, I needed to develop a standard protocol of practice by distilling my theoretical knowledge and clinical experience into patterns and rules of diagnosis and treatment. Only then would I be able to apply classical medicine to a modern context. I began to seek the patterns and internal logic of formula architecture based on the assumption that most effective Chinese medicine derives from combinations of formulas. This was my third period of study. This line of inquiry would not only open up new ways of thinking about treating certain diseases, it would also deepen and strengthen the theory of differential diagnosis.

Reading Chen Xiu-yuan's "10 Recommendations"

1. Chen Xiu-yuan states that "Zhong-jing compiled the formulas of Master Yi (Yi Yin) and other formulas passed down from antiquity in the *Treatise on Cold Damage* and the *Essential Prescriptions of the Golden Cabinet*" thus, "my first recommendation is to read the works of Zhong-jing."

2. Chen Believed that modern practitioners needed to recognize the negative influence wrought on Chinese medicine by the four masters of the Jin and Yuan Dynasties.[27] They "claimed to be pragmatic and straightforward practitioners of the essentials of the medicine" but were in fact sophists and "despite claiming to respect Zhong-jing in name, they rarely provided commentary on his work or showed how to use it in practice. Even worse, they stood truth on its head, making the misguided claim that Zhong-jing's works were only applicable to cold damage and Gui Zhi and Ma Huang were only useful in northern climates or in winter." Practitioners that had been influenced by their mistaken views had to disabuse themselves of such notions. Thus, his second recommendation was "know where one has erred and take steps to improve."

3. Chen thought that, "Except in chronic diseases, most formulas should take effect from the first to the fourth dose." He claimed that jīngfāng formulas should have a near "instantaneous effect". The *Inner Canon* states, "After one packet, it should be clear if the right formula was used. After two packets, the disease should be

---

[27] Liu Wan-su (劉完素), Zhang Cong-zheng (張從正), Li Gao or Li Dong-yuan (李杲), Zhu Zhen-heng or Zhu Dan-xi (朱震亨)

resolved" and "the disease should be resolved as soon as the formula is consumed." The *Treatise* also states, "If the illness resolves after the first dose, there is no need to drink the rest of the decoction from the first packet." Thus, Chen's third recommendation was "modern practitioners must recognize that jīngfāng formulas should have a rapid effect."

4. Chen believed that the main key to *Treatise* formulas was "preservation of fluid". Both Gui Zhi Tang and Ma Huang Tang, Chen said, "were designed to preserve fluid". As for *Essential Prescriptions* formulas, "most are guided by a warm supplementing formula design". "Later commentators did not understand and were rigid in their thinking." Thus, Chen's fourth recommendation is to "understand the strengths and weaknesses of jīngfāng."

5. Chen argued that modern practitioners were unclear about the dosages in the *Treatise*. In his fifth recommendation he states: "They fear the doses are too high and don't dare use them. Yet, they fail to realize that materia medica lost its way in the Song and Yuan dynasties and fell into extreme disrepair in the Ming dynasty with Li Shi-zhen (李時珍).

6. Chen wrote: "Whether in cold damage, miscellaneous disease, or diseases of the yáng or yīn channels, as long as the disease involves disharmony of construction and defense, Gui Zhi Tang will resolve it perfectly. Likewise, in diseases where evil qì cannot pivot outwards, Xiao Chai Hu Tang will completely resolve them." As such, Chen's sixth recommendation was, "learning how to use these two formulas should be the foundation of every physician's practice."

7. Chen argued that in emergency situations, practitioners shouldn't just rely on Ren Shen. He believed that in life-or-death situations, "One should still use Zhong-jing's methodologies, returning yáng with Si Ni Tang and Bai Tong Tang, preserving fluid with Bai Hu

Tang or Cheng Qi Tang, assisting pivoting and transformation, harmonizing the organs and bowels, all with attention to the state of stomach qì."

8. Chen stated: "The more one reads Zhong-jing's works, the more they resonate. The more one uses his formulas, the more miraculous they seem. After using jīngfāng in clinic, I often go over Zhong-jing's works at night and come to many fascinating insights. Thus, my eighth recommendation is to review the classics to gain new insights."

9. "Zhong-jing's stature in the Chinese medical tradition is similar to the canonized greats of the Confucian tradition. Those who expound and propagate his works respect this tradition, while those that run contrary to his ideas are heretical to this tradition." Various post-classical physicians made certain trifling achievements, but they cannot be viewed in the same category as Zhong-jing. If students fail to set a firm foundation in the *Treatise* and the *Essential Prescriptions*, they are liable to be misguided by post-classical theory. Thus, Chen's ninth recommendation was to "focus on jīngfāng in one's studies".

10. Chen encouraged practitioners to be forthright in their interactions with each other. He thought that this was the only way that the writings of Qi Bo, Huang Di and Zhong-jing could be fully clarified and expounded. Insofar as he believed that practitioners should speak openly and frankly among themselves, his tenth recommendation was to "not hide anything in one's conversation with other practitioners and to be cordial and respectful in interactions."

It took me some time, but after many years I finally gained a clear understanding of this chapter. When I read this chapter, it feels as if I'm having a conversation with Chen Xiu-yuan himself. Reading this essay helped me realize that Chinese medicinal knowledge is not only applicable in clinic, it has a much wider scope of application, including what is now known as Chinese medical psychology and Chinese medical sociology. Ultimately, of course, these other fields must also be applied to clinical practice to improve our diagnostics and treatment outcomes.

Chinese Doctors Should Not Indulge in Extremism

Tōdō Yoshimasu believed that six-conformation theory was not included in the original *Treatise on Cold Damage* text and was inserted later by scholars from the *Inner Canon* school of thought. Due to this belief, he promoted the practice of removing all such theory from the *Treatise* and leaving only formulas and patterns. Thus, his book *The Categorized Formulas* did just that, and advanced the notion of "using the formulas and herbs that fit the pattern, which is the practice of formula and herb pattern correspondence." Lu Yuan-lei once wrote: "Certain old tomes state 'Xiao Chai Hu Tang treats shàoyáng disease, evil lodged in the half interior half exterior, fullness and discomfort in the chest and rib-side, alternating heat effusion and cold aversion, vexation, nausea and a wiry and thin pulse'. Why do they bother to complicate things by writing 'evil lodged in the half interior half exterior'?" This kind of polemic is a bit extreme and he was later attacked by many in the Chinese medicine community and ended up being something of a failure.

What the Chinese medicine world needs now is more practitioners like Huang Huang (黃煌) who dare to question, dare to experiment, dare to seek the truth and dare to innovate. We need practitioners like Huang Huang who are steeped in the classics, willing to lead and set an example, seek truth from facts, and yet are measured in their statements and do not indulge in extremism.

Modern Chinese Doctors Should Have a Good Knowledge of Western Medicine

I once had a 30-year-old patient arrive at my clinic with abdominal pain. He related that the pain had begun the previous night after drinking too much and he had sought treatment from one Dr. Lin Hua-qing. Dr. Lin noted that the patient presented with heat effusion, a temperature of 38°C, bitterness of the mouth and halitosis, upper-abdominal pain, restricted and tight feeling in upper abdomen, nausea, vomiting, and occasional spasming in the arms and legs. The pulse was slippery and rapid, and the tongue was red with a yellow, greasy coating. The patient noted that he had found a roundworm in his vomit. Dr. Lin diagnosed this as middle burner damp-heat, liver qì stagnation transforming to heat and attacking the stomach, replete congestion of heat toxins, and roundworms harassing upwards. His treatment was to course the liver, unblock the interior, purge downwards, quicken the blood and dispel stasis, descend counterflow and abate pain, and dispel roundworms. He prescribed Da Chai Hu Tang plus Mang Xiao, Gui Zhi, Chuan Jiao, Huang Lian, Wu Mei, Xi Xin etc. The patient continually asked Dr. Lin what was wrong with him, but Dr. Lin couldn't provide a western medical diagnosis, saying only that it was a GI tract issue. Dr. Lin was a Chinese medicine practitioner of the old school. He had studied some Western medicine here and there, but never systematically. This kind of situation might be awkward, but it is a fairly common or normal occurrence for Chinese medical doctors. However, the patient just wouldn't let it go—he was dissatisfied with Dr. Lin's ambiguous answer and asked: "Well where exactly in my GI system is the problem?" Dr. Lin just lacked the knowledge to say what the precise disease name was for this patient's problem, so he answered: "Don't concern yourself with where the disease is located. Just decoct the herbs that I gave you and your abdominal pain will probably resolve."

The patient took the prescription from the clinic pharmacy and headed home, but he was still feeling hesitant about Dr. Lin's diagnosis, and he was still having intermittent bouts of abdominal pain, so he decided to go to a western clinic instead of going home and taking the herbs. Based upon the patient's history of gall stones, alcohol abuse, and overeating, along with the heat effusion, upper abdomen pain, nausea, vomiting, and restricted band-like feeling in the upper abdomen, the western doctor diagnosed him with acute pancreatitis. The spasms in the arms and legs, which Dr. Lin had diagnosed as "liver fire transforming to wind", were diagnosed by the western doctor as hypocalcemia. To the patient, these were two completely irreconcilable diagnoses. The western doctor told the patient that spasming in acute pancreatitis was a sign of severe disease and had a poor prognosis. As such, the doctor summoned an ambulance, and the patient was taken to a local city hospital for immediate emergency treatment. To mitigate the abdominal pain, nausea and vomiting, the doctor needled the patient with a 3 cun needle at a sensitive spot below GB34. Only seconds later, the patient reported a substantial mitigation of symptoms. The doctor continued to twist, lift, and thrust the needle to stimulate the point every five minutes. By the time the ambulance arrived, the patient was already feeling substantially more comfortable. He continually praised the western doctor's treatment and was deeply dissatisfied with what he perceived to be Dr. Lin's negligence.

At the hospital, the patient was again diagnosed with acute pancreatitis and given a range of treatments, but nothing seemed to improve his condition. With no other choices left, the attending doctor called in a doctor from the Chinese medicine department. The doctor told the patient that the western doctors had made the correct diagnosis, that their treatments had all been necessary and proper, and they had paved the way for Chinese medicine to be effective. Like Dr. Lin, the Chinese doctor diagnosed the patient with middle burner damp-heat, liver fire attacking the stomach, and replete heat engendering wind. He prescribed one packet of Qing Yi Tang[28] and told the patient he didn't need to refrain from eating, could take out the feeding tube, and could stop taking Atropine. After taking the herbs, the patient passed a large amount of turbid, malodorous stools, after which his condition notably improved. Even the western medical team had to admit that of all the interventions, Qing Yi Tang had been the most effective. The patient realized that the formula he'd taken was similar to the one Dr. Lin had prescribed, so he continued by taking Dr. Lin's formula and his condition improved even more. However, he still didn't understand why the western medical interventions had failed even when their diagnosis was accurate and why did Dr. Lin's formula work even though he didn't know the western medical diagnosis? After he made a complete recovery, he went to see Dr. Lin again and put these two questions to him. Dr. Lin just sighed and seemed to be unable to answer his questions. He ultimately made the painful realization that his lack of western medical knowledge was holding him back as a Chinese medical clinician.

This acute pancreatitis case study once again demonstrates the strengths and weaknesses of Chinese and Western medicine. Chinese medical physicians must have a good knowledge of Western medicine. That is to say, in order to provide a better service for patients, it is important that Chinese doctors have a good grasp of western medical diagnosis and treatment skills.

This is a topic worthy of deeper exploration. Let us frame this discussion around the differing theoretical models represented by western and Chinese medicine.

In Western medicine, it is believed that pancreatitis is mainly caused by unregulated activation of trypsin, which then auto-digests the gland. As such, inhibiting excretion and activation of trypsin can stop or mitigate the progress of the disease. This is the main objective of western medical treatment, and all other interventions, such as fasting, intubation, and atropine injection all revolve around it. The point is to use every means possible to suppress the physiological and pathological

---

[28]"Clear Pancreas Decoction": Chai Hu 15g, Bai Shao 15g, Da Huang 15g, Huang Qin 9g, Hu Huang Lian 9g, Mu Xiang 9g, Yan Hu Suo 9g, Mang Xiao 9g (quite similar to Dr. Lin's formula)

functioning of the gastrointestinal system, to allow the digestive system to "calm down". By contrast, ancient Chinese medicine's approach to acute abdominal pain is "supplement vacuity and purge repletion." In replete acute abdominal pain, the treatment method is to "unblock the painful area and open up the congested region". In vacuous acute abdominal pain, the treatment aims to "supplement vacuity" and "treat the stopped by stopping". In terms of jīngfāng formula patterns, acute abdominal pain is usually treated with Da Huang family formulas such as Da Xian Xiong Tang, Cheng Qi Tang formulas, and Da Chai Hu Tang, Bai Shao family formulas such as Gui Zhi Jia Shao Yao Tang, Xiao Jian Zhong Tang, and Da Jian Zhong Tang and Fu Zi family formulas such as Shao Yao Gan Cao Fu Zi Tang and Fu Zi Jing Mi Tang. Of course, Chinese medicine does not have the medical term "acute pancreatitis" and doesn't have the language to describe its etiology from a western medical perspective. That being said, the symptomatology of this kind of condition has been well known since antiquity and the understanding of the progression of this disease and corresponding treatment strategy is quite mature in Chinese medicine. Of course, the strategy in question is not oriented towards a single disease and is certainly not designed to treat acute pancreatitis specifically. What modern medicine fails to realize is that the strategy to which I'm referring is a systematic protocol for the treatment of all disease. It can be used for any disease, and so of course it can also be used for acute pancreatitis. The inception, progression, and prognosis for acute pancreatitis can all be understood through the three yīn three yáng system of the *Treatise on Cold Damage*. Indeed, Dr. Lin diagnosed the patient with a shàoyáng-yángmíng Da Chai Hu Tang formula pattern. Because Juéyīn and shàoyáng are an interior-exterior pair, it was to be expected that the patient might present with certain Juéyīn symptoms like roundworms "harassing upwards" and "arm and leg spasms". Dr. Lin's prescription of Da Chai Hu Tang plus (half of) Wu Mei Wan was a perfectly suitable formula for the patient's presentation and was no less legitimate than the hospital doctor's prescription of Qing Yi Tang. Additionally, this formula was entirely consistent with the Chinese medical principles of "unblock the painful area" and "open up congestion" used in treatment of replete acute abdominal pain. The opening, unblocking, and purging approach in Chinese medicine for the treatment of replete acute abdominal pain is the complete opposite of Western medicine's repressing and inhibiting approach. As for which approach is better, the results of the above case should make the answer abundantly clear.

That being said, we should remember that vacuous patterns can also present with acute abdominal conditions. Various *kampo* practitioners have given detailed discussions of the involvement of Gui Zhi Jia Shao Yao Tang, Shao Yao Gan Cao Fu Zi Tang, Fu Zi Jing Mi Tang, Xiao Jian Zhong Tang, and Da Jian Zhong Tang formula patterns in acute abdominal conditions. Additionally, they have used these formulas extensively to treat related diseases with excellent results. We mustn't ignore the fantastic contributions of Japanese *kampo* practitioners to the jīngfāng lineage and should strive to learn more from their experience. In sum, the jīngfāng approach to the treatment of acute abdominal conditions is based on pattern differentiation, while the western medical approach is plagued by certain blind spots and biases.

Western medical abdominal assessment can determine the degree of liver cirrhosis just based on palpation. If the liver feels like palpation of the forehead, this is considered "hard". If it feels like the tip of the nose, this is considered "moderate hardness" and if it feels like the lips, it's considered "soft".

A patient that often coughs up pink-red, foamy phlegm suddenly awakes in the night with a suffocating and panicked feeling that lasts for 30 seconds or longer before slowly abating. How should such a patient be diagnosed and treated? This is a clear indicator of left heart failure with pulmonary edema that you would only know if you were to study Western medicine. Modern Chinese doctors must acquire this type of knowledge. This knowledge will not only help you frame treatment, it will also help you maintain your status of medical authority in the eyes of your patients. In these modern times, if a doctor lacks even this basic diagnostic ability, they will surely lose the trust of their patients.

Patient-Based Treatment Sets
Chinese Medicine Apart

Kampo physicians have a much different conception of Chinese medical disease names than the common paradigm in China's Chinese medical circles. They are vehemently opposed to any approach that takes a disease name as the target of treatment. For instance, Keisetsu Ōtsuka argued: "Chinese medicine is not like Western medicine, wherein once one has determined the disease, the treatment strategy automatically follows based on protocol. In Chinese medicine, the diagnosis and treatment strategy are based on the patient's condition, pulse, and constitution. Because patients are used to getting a disease name as a diagnosis from western doctors, we too must appease them with a diagnosis, but this should not be the focus of treatment. Disease names are written in books but don't exist in the actual world, what actually exists is the patient. It would be highly unsuitable to treat a living, breathing patient, with all the specificity and uniqueness of their condition based upon a rigid protocol for one abstract and non-existent disease name. On this point we are quite clear: there is no such thing as disease that exists independently from the patient." If we as physicians do not have access to a patient's presentation, we cannot talk in the abstract about how to treat them. When speaking about bronchial asthma approaches, we are not referring to a set protocol, but rather just generally discussing certain patterns that appear in bronchial asthma more frequently in clinic. This is entirely different from how Western medicine has a set protocol for the treatment of bronchial asthma. Ōtsuka summed up his point on this question, saying: "Patient-Based Treatment is What Sets Chinese Medicine Apart".

Treating Cancer with Chinese Medicine

There is no question that Chinese medicine is an extremely valuable modality in the treatment of cancer and that jīngfāng medicine's formula pattern correspondence approach can produce particularly impressive results. That said, Chinese physicians should be clear on one point when it comes to the treatment of cancer: In the early and middle stages of treatment, the standard of success should be measured by the patient's overall health and sense of well-being, their vital signs, and routine exam results as opposed to oncology blood test or biopsy results. If one overly focuses on these results, treatment will likely be abandoned halfway. The proper approach to treatment should not be based on the disease itself and there shouldn't be an expectation of a linear path to recovery.

So how specifically should one approach the treatment of cancer using jīngfāng medicine's formula pattern correspondence? While every situation will be different, the imperative of this approach is to identify the key pattern and prescribe based upon formula pattern correspondence. If the patient has recalcitrant heat effusion, the focus of treatment should be on "heat effusion" as the key pattern and one should seek the proper formula pattern corresponding to the patient's presentation, whether it be a Gui Zhi Tang, Ma Huang Tang, Xiao Chai Hu Tang, Bai Hu Tang, Cheng Qi Tang, or Si Ni Tang formula pattern.

In the acute phase of a patient's cancer condition, it is inadvisable to add herbs aimed directly at addressing the tumor. These can be added once the patient's condition is stable.

As long as the cancer patient still has some traces of cancer left in their body, they will likely have certain symptoms and signs. The focus of our treatment should be on the patient's most pressing symptom at any stage of their condition, always performing formula pattern correspondence at each stage based on the patient's key pattern. For instance, if the patient's heat effusion abates and they develop diarrhea, we should pivot to finding a formula pattern to match this new key symptom of diarrhea such as Ge Gen Tang, Ge Gen Qin Lian Tang, Huang Qin Tang, Ban Xia Xie Xin Tang, Li Zhong Tang, Si Ni Tang, or Wu Mei Wan. This process takes time, patience, and wisdom.

The Spark of Zhong-jing's Art is Being Rekindled in China

Yue Mei-zhong, Liu Du-zhou, Hu Xi-shu, and Huang Huang are all jīng-fāng practitioners, but their specific approaches vary widely. I'm often asked to clarify the difference between Huang Huang and Hu Xi-shu's "formula pattern diagnosis" approach and Liu Du-zhou and Yue Mei-zhong's mechanism-based diagnosis approach.

The difference between these two camps is an objective reality—in the Chinese medicine world, there is no lack of debate between various lineages and each lineage seems to have its own unassailable logic. According to my limited knowledge, I believe that the "formula pattern diagnosis" school's emphasis on "formula pattern correspondence" is preferable to an emphasis on mechanism-based diagnosis and treatment. I believe that an emphasis on "analysis of constitution" is preferable to an "analysis of etiology and pathomechanism". I believe emphasizing "sole adherence to the approaches of Zhong-jing" is preferable to an "ecumenical" approach. I believe emphasizing "the importance of studying *kampo*" is preferable to "learning from each and every school". I believe that emphasizing "study of common western diseases treated by each formula pattern" is preferable to "study of Chinese and western disease names". I believe emphasis on "holistic treatment" is preferable to "specialization". I believe emphasizing "abdominal palpation and abdominal patterns" is preferable to emphasis on "pulse patterns and pulse diagnosis". I believe that emphasizing an approach marked by "proceeding from medicinals, to formulas, to methods to principles" is preferable to "proceeding from principles, to methods, to formulas to medicinals". These beliefs, which are all representative of the "formula pattern diagnosis", are in stark opposition to traditional mainstream Chinese medicine.

In my opinion, the "mechanism-based diagnosis" approach of Yue Mei-zhong and Liu Du-zhou represents the mainstream paradigm of modern Chinese medicine. This approach is suitable for physicians with a strong foundation in Chinese medical theory who wish to prioritize theory over clinic. It is an approach that might be suitably adopted by those going into the academic study of Chinese medicine. The "formula pattern diagnosis" approach promoted by Huang Huang and Hu Xi-shu is still in a formative, inchoate stage — this diagnostic system is not complete, it cannot be applied in all situations and, as Huang Huang says, "we can only seek truth, not totality". That being said, formula pattern diagnosis has already proven to be a vital method in clinic with unlimited potential for development. It is a quick and simple method to achieve proficiency in clinic. Huang Huang's approach has become a guiding light for young students entering into the study of jīngfāng. Huang Huang's system in particular has an irreplaceable value in the context of the modern ideological zeitgeist. I often read through his books and experience, time and again, the untold pleasure of reading. When I read his works, it is as if the nourishing and inspiring achievements of Chinese medical history are being reenacted and embodied all around me. As a clinical Chinese doctor, I wish to offer my respect and admiration to Dr. Huang Huang for all that he has contributed.

Zhang Tai-yan's lament that Zhong-jing's art was only truly being practiced in the east (Japan) is slowly becoming a footnote of history. Through the work of Hu Xi-shu, Huang Huang, and their promotion of formula pattern diagnosis, the spark of Zhong-jing's art is being rekindled in China.

Editor's Post-Script

Wenzhou, a land traversed by rivers and bordered by mountains and ocean, is a bustling and beautiful southern city which boasts both a deep, traditional cultural heritage, and a youthful vitality. In this wondrous country, an army of Chinese medical doctors work with quiet determination to uphold the great Chinese medical foundation of Wenzhou and maintain the health of her people. Among them are elite scholars pursuing bold lines of medical research as well as clinicians with extraordinary skills from countless lineages. This is a place where masters of the craft lay hidden in plain sight everywhere one looks, unassumingly plying their trades in hospitals, county health centers, and quiet village clinics throughout the city. Lou Shao-kun is well-known as one of the greats among this elite corps of physicians. Enduring extremely difficult circumstances, he taught himself Chinese medicine through a process of tireless study, laboring day by day in practice and research to become a consummate practitioner and famous physician of the jīngfāng tradition.

In the early summer of 2012, we members of the editing team had the distinct pleasure of meeting Dr. Lou for the first time at the launch of his autobiography, "A Life Devoted to Chinese Medicine". Dr. Lou was a man of deep cultural cultivation with a distinctive flare to his speech and a soft, mellifluous Zhe-jiang accent that was both inviting and endearing. He exuded the temperament and disposition of a classic southern intellectual. Whenever he spoke about Chinese medicine or jīngfāng, he became particularly animated and effusive, and his enthusiasm was contagious. The crowd was packed to the doors at the Xinhua Bookstore for the launch of Lou's autobiography and the 100 or so books they prepared for sale were signed and sold in a matter of minutes. We were amazed at the reception Dr. Lou received and to this day it has left a deep impression on us.

Dr. Lou is now over seventy-years-old, but he still keeps up a frenetic pace of clinical practice, academic research, self-study, lecturing, and online engagements. Propelled by his undeviating love for jīngfāng he tirelessly travels throughout the country, spreading his medical knowledge within China and abroad, accumulating an increasingly thick oeuvre of medical treatises and case studies. Dr. Lou's daughter, Dr. Lou Shen-shan meticulously compiled Dr. Lou's writings into two volumes (*Dr. Lou Shao Kun's Case Studies and Medical Treatises* and *Dr. Lou Shaokun's Lectures on Jīngfāng*) and submitted them to us for editing. We were honored to receive these writings from Dr. Lou and felt a great sense of responsibility to make sure they were transmitted faithfully. Dr. Lou's writing is a true reflection of his character—a practical and familiar prose style with a unique individual flair, these two volumes are filled with his distinctive clinical experiences and insights and feature clear articulations of his various theories that reflect a deep cultural cultivation and rock-solid foundation in clinical and theoretical medical knowledge. It was a true pleasure to edit Dr. Lou's writings and we all could sense the passion and commitment to the everyday clinical practice of jīngfāng which shines through his writings. We know that the practical, in-clinic feel of these writings with their direct insights and unfiltered experience will be a major boon to students and practitioners of jīngfāng.

The jīngfāng lineage, and indeed, the Chinese medical profession as a whole, needs many more practitioners like Dr. Lou.

—August 16th, 2018

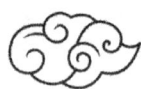